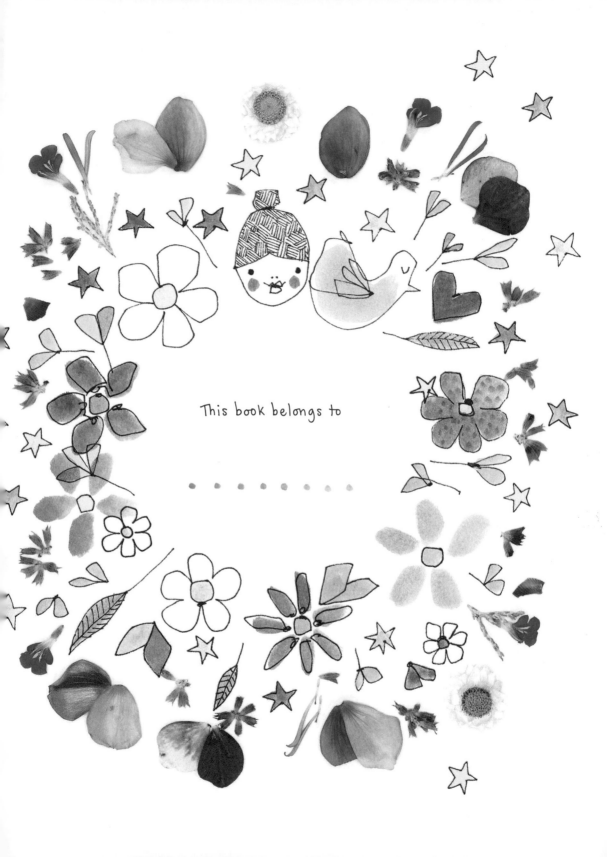

This book belongs to

· · · · · · · · ·

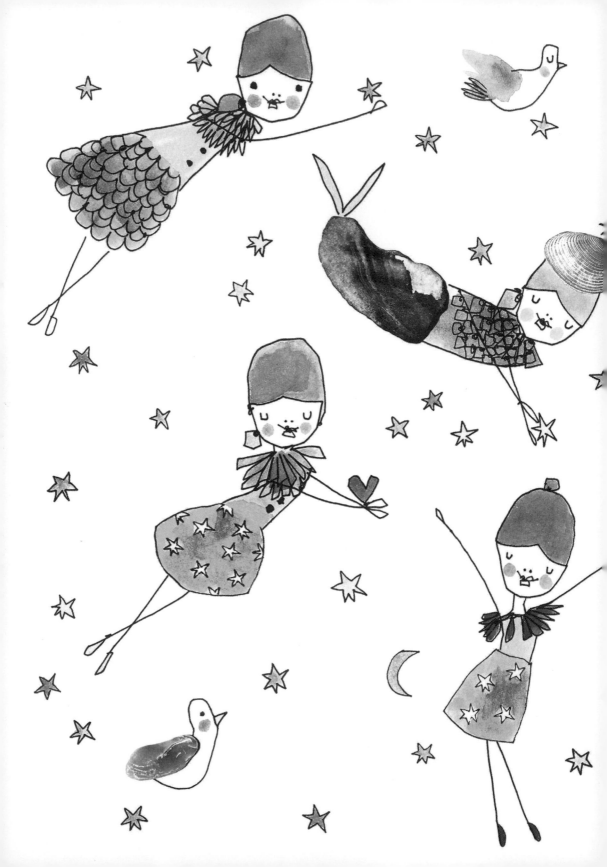

FIND YOUR SPARKLE

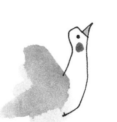

Meredith Gaston

Hardie Grant

BOOKS

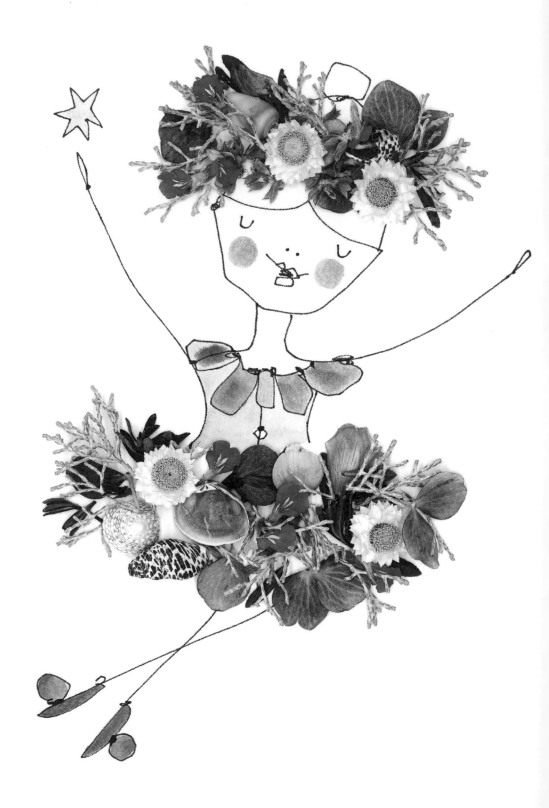

All things by immortal power

Near or far,

Hiddenly

To each other linked are,

That thou canst not stir a flower

Without troubling of a star.

Francis Thompson

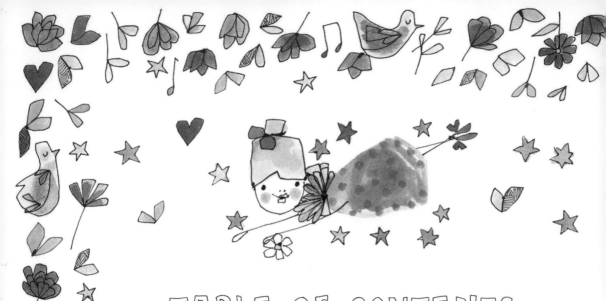

TABLE OF CONTENTS

Dearest Reader 2

Enjoying this Book 5

EXPLORING YOUR SPARKLE 11

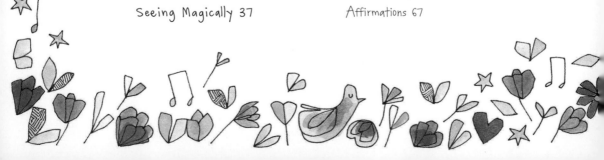

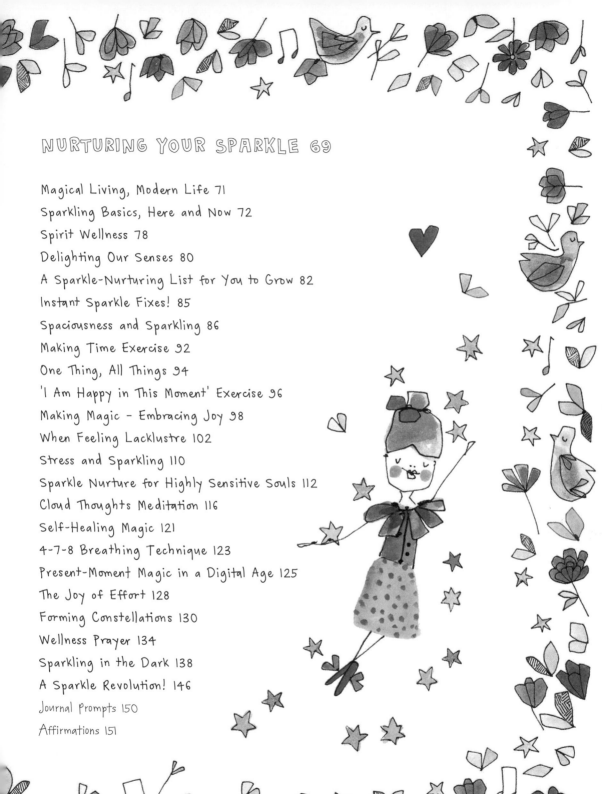

NURTURING YOUR SPARKLE 69

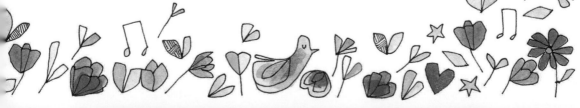

NOURISHING YOUR SPARKLE 153

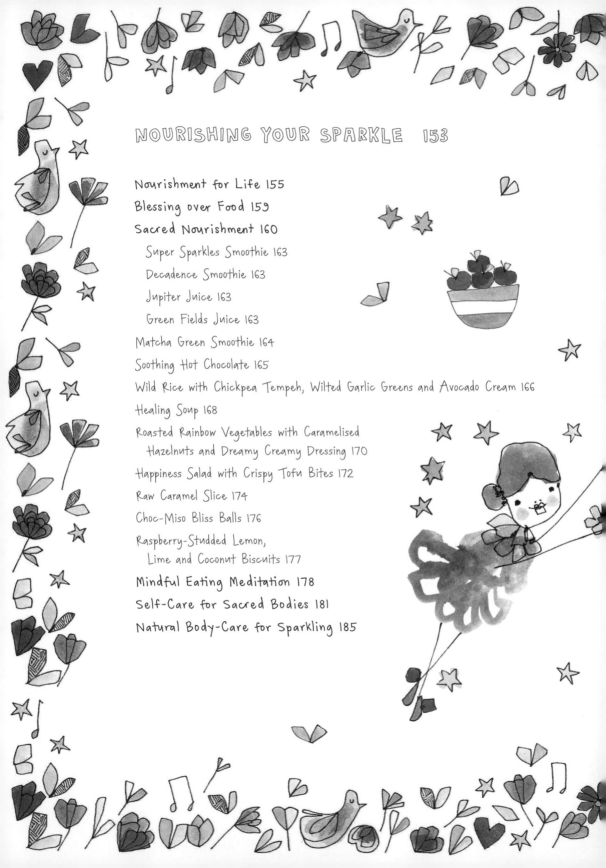

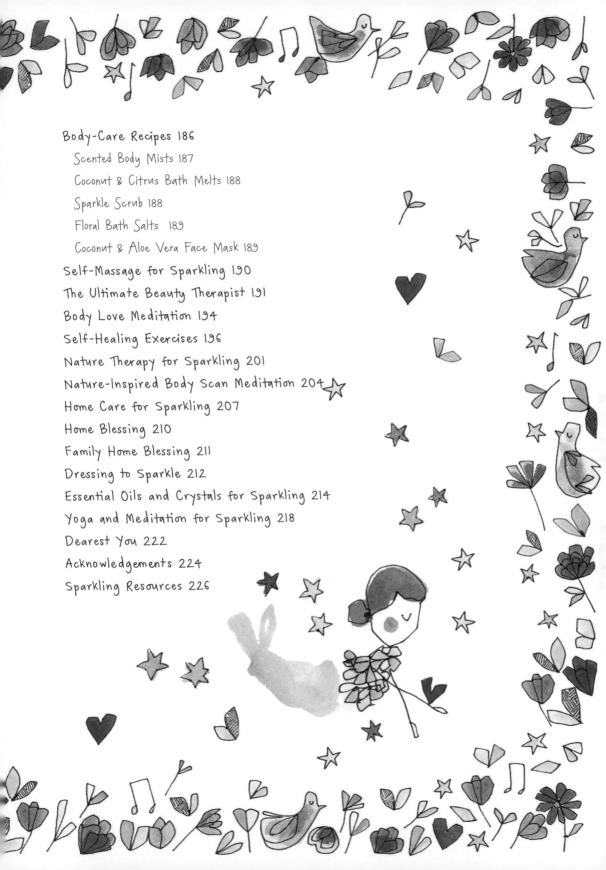

CLOSE YOUR
EYES AND
FALL IN LOVE.
STAY THERE.

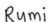

Rumi

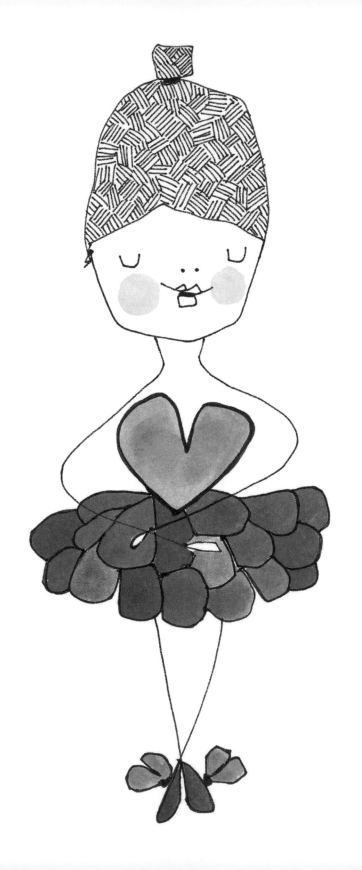

DEAREST READER,

This is a love letter to your spirit . . . the rose in your cheek, the twinkle in your eye and the spring in your step. It is a jubilant ode to the magical, timeless part within you that sparkles with life and hums in tune with all creation; lovingly woven from the same cloth as the earth, the sea and the sky, all creatures great and small.

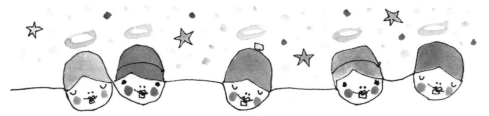

Indeed, we human beings contain all the energy, mystery and magic of the universe within us, imbuing us with infinite creativity, inspiration and vitality. We all too often simply forget that such beauty and wisdom dances effortlessly within us, glistening, wild and free. While we might look in many places for happiness, we already possess the magic we seek. It belongs to us as a luminous, ever-present sparkle within us: a precious kind of energy that we are invited to explore, nurture and nourish each day of our lives.

Nurturing our inner sparkle is a joyous practice especially worthy of our devotion, time and care. By tending lovingly to our spirits and inviting them to guide us, we awaken to the magic and beauty of living. While caring for our bodies and the physical world around us is very important, caring for our inner world is essential for our lifelong joy and vitality.

Life calls us to nourish our spirits with tenderness and delight each step of the way. Any small, tender act of self-care – a deep breath, an early night, a life-giving meal, or a slow potter in nature – can nourish, restore and reignite our inner glow. A faithful guiding light, our inner sparkle flickers when we need to rest and gives us encouraging little signs when we soothe and care for ourselves. It dims when we ignore the calls of our hearts, and glistens brightly when we craft courageous, intuitive lives from our truest values and dreams. Attuning to our inner sparkle awakens us to the deepest kind of wisdom, love and inspiration we could ever know.

While we may look very different from one another on the outside and lead unique, separate-looking lives, what we all have in common is our shared aliveness. Our collective human being-ness. It is this spiritual essence within us that we recognise in each other, especially in our kindest, most unguarded and tender moments. Sensing the sublime and timeless connection between ourselves and all others with whom we share our world, we may draw boundless compassion and energy from our shared story. We may open our hearts at last to the meaning, purpose and belonging for which we all inherently yearn. We are deeply creative, imaginative beings, far more powerful and magical than we realise. When we find our heaven within us, we may find it in one another and in our world at large. One by one as we nurture and share our sparkles, we form healing constellations that illuminate our world.

It is an exciting time to be alive now as, in my eyes, our world is changing. We are looking to exchange tiresome comparison, competition and clutter for meaningful collaboration, connection and compassion. We see that by elevating others, we too sparkle more brightly. Tired of jam-packed agendas, burdensome hurries and worries, we are seeking greater inspiration, spaciousness and happiness in our days. We yearn to touch the kinds of sublime experiences that inspire our curiosity, playfulness and wonder, encouraging us to believe in bliss on earth. We long to experience our lives not as problems to be solved but as soulful, joyous, unfolding adventures; creative journeys through which we awaken, grow and blossom. It cannot be forgotten that we human beings are crafted of ancient stardust and other miracles, and by no mistake either. We are here to find our sparkle.

May you feel encouraged to live each day to the fullest, never letting the beauty of your life pass you by. May you choose to see the magic in life and, in doing so, let your life become infinitely more magical. May the divine inner sparkle within you feel uplifted, enchanted and inspired.

Love, Meredith X

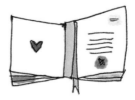

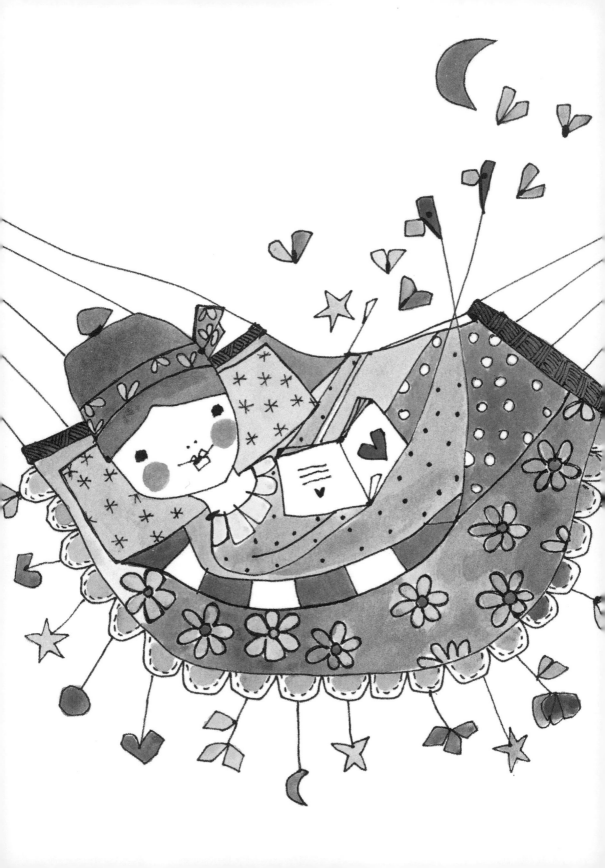

ENJOYING THIS BOOK

This book is divided into three sections: Exploring Your Sparkle,
Nurturing Your Sparkle and Nourishing Your Sparkle. It is a book to
be taken in slowly and deeply over time. Open to any page for a dose
of sparkling inspiration, or savour it from cover to cover. Feel encouraged
to underline or highlight passages that ignite your sparkle, and let the
words and pictures spring into your heart. This book is a joyous, open
invitation to explore the lightness of being, to courageously satisfy your
hunger for life in nurturing ways that allow your spirit to blossom.

In the first section we will look at what it means to sparkle: what it might look like and
how it might feel. Gather inspiration to write or rewrite your own story, dipping into
the joy and creativity on offer to you simply by choosing to see through loving, curious
and appreciative eyes. Feel inspired to go within and draw from the infinite wellspring of
creativity and wisdom that you possess. Indeed, simply by existing we are all organically
part of a delightful, mysterious and empowering intelligence. There is so much more to
life than meets our eyes, and an entire universe of enchanting, guiding wonders simply
waiting for us to suspend our disbelief and tune into it!

In the second section of this book, Nurturing Your Sparkle, we will discover practical
ways in which we can cultivate and maintain a sense of joyous wellbeing in daily life.
We will look at self-care practices involving our thoughts and mindset, emotional
intelligence, the energy of our physical bodies, and the desires of our unique spirits.
By embracing our authentic and whole selves, living with intention and joy, we are
able to sparkle for ourselves while being lighthouses for others. We become kinder,
happier, healthier, more compassionate people who can contribute to the greater good.
We awaken to our own potential, the potential of life and each other.

In this bountiful second section we will also explore the various shared human experiences in busy modern life that are urging us to shift by discovering and harnessing our innate magnificence and magic. Explore and grow your own self-motivating, self-healing and creative powers. Cultivate courage and integrity by crafting a life in tune with the truest desires of your spirit. Discover simple, daily ways of embracing the magic of life: ways that help you to harmonise your inner and outer worlds, that balance rest and play, and that honour your innermost sparkle.

In section three, Nourishing Your Sparkle, we draw on ancient wisdom to help us flourish in our modern world. Nourishing our sparkle reconnects us with ourselves and our earth, allowing us to experience true pleasure, peace and fulfilment in our days. This section is brimming with prompts and activities, nourishing recipes, rituals and inspirations to encourage and uplift you. Discover edible earthy delights, guided mindfulness exercises and exciting, natural beauty secrets.

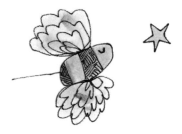

The words 'spirit' and 'spiritual' can possess esoteric and, for some of us, religious connotations. They might even be words that make some of us feel uncomfortable. And yet, here we are, spirits having a human experience! Our spirits are self-sown seeds of a higher intelligence of which we are all a part, and in which we exist in accordance with a perfect, natural law.

The miraculous nature of our consciousness, minds and bodies is so often taken for granted. In this luscious and creative third section, we redirect our attention back to our spirits. Back to nature and our earth, and back to the soothing, enriching and energising benefits that wonder, faith and gratitude bring.

Savouring the Mindfulness Exercises, Soul-Food Recipes and Journal Prompts Within

I hope you will enjoy the various mindfulness exercises throughout this book. They have been created especially for you as you commit to exploring and nurturing your own inner sparkle. The activities in this book are simple and joyous techniques to still and quieten your mind when needed, or to stimulate freshness and energy when required. May you be encouraged to carve out the sacred space and time you need in your life to know and care for yourself deeply.

The journal prompts in this book have been written to stimulate you and encourage you to put pen to paper. There is a certain magical power in putting pen to paper. We materialise abstract thoughts by putting them into written words, welcoming self-expression while inviting greater insight and clarity. With our words we may be honest and courageous, intimate and free. We may begin to turn our dreams into realities and document our wonderful journeys. Please use the journal prompts within to connect with your spirit. Choose a journal or notebook that you love and, once you finish it, treasure it and find another. Keep writing. Keep documenting and celebrating all the days of your life. Our journals are places for good days and hard days, for moments of joy and moments of challenge. Creating a journalling practice is a gift, and a daily ritual that can be savoured for life. I write morning and night and love the comforting, steady rhythm this brings to my days. However you please, put pen to paper and embrace the therapeutic and magical benefits.

I see positive affirmations as powerful statements of truth to uplift, inspire and transform us. Our thoughts create our worlds. When we take care of our thoughts, we take care of our whole lives. May the affirmations within this book inspire you on your way as you embrace the magic of living. May they also encourage you to create your own affirmations – ones that you can write, draw, think, sing and dance about. Statements of truth that resonate with you and support you to experience greater bliss, freedom and wellbeing in your life.

In section three you will find various exercises to explore your creativity and nourish your imagination. These exercises can be enjoyed at your own pace, in your own space and time, and with any additional flourishes you desire. Be free, and allow the joyous unfolding of the creative process to be your destination.

I love to cook with fresh, organic, local and seasonal ingredients. Eating like this is a wonderful way to celebrate real food, connect with the earth, and cultivate sparkling health. Wherever possible, source your ingredients as thoughtfully as you can and eat with gratitude and pleasure.

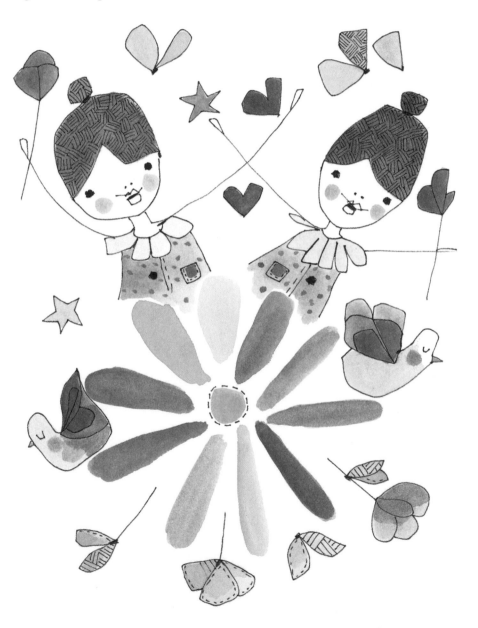

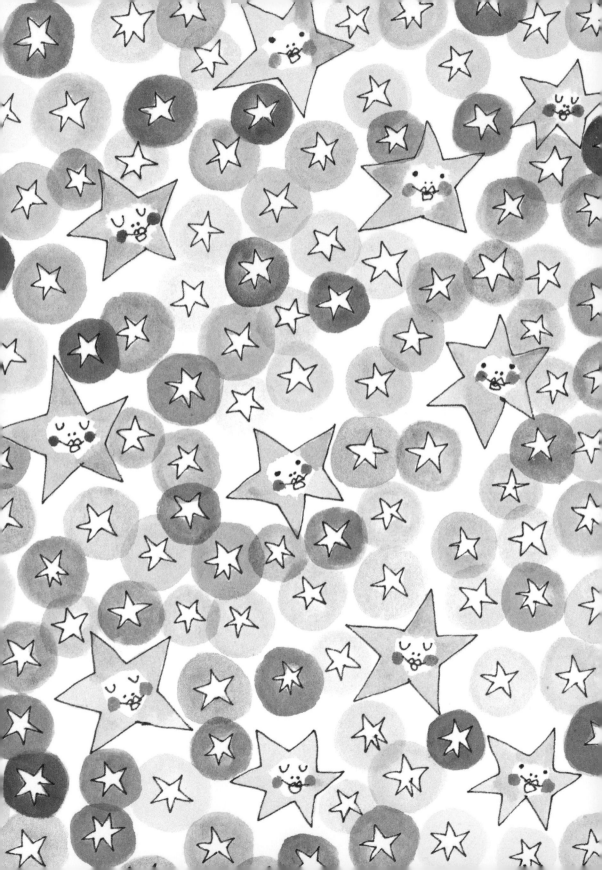

EXPLORING YOUR SPARKLE

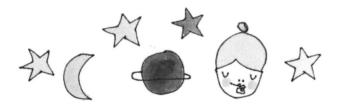

Let's delve deeper into exploring the divine inner sparkle we all possess, connecting us to a bigger picture of love and life.

While we talk daily about self-care including the ways we move, eat, drink, think and sleep, we rarely speak directly to the wellness of our spirits. Understanding and caring for ourselves as spiritual beings radically shifts our sense of self, time and space, and inspires renewed gratitude and wonder for life. At spirit level we can truly assess our priorities and sense of purpose, moving in the direction of true peace and joy.

Disconnected from the calls of our spirits, we will always sense that something is missing in our lives. As if we lack something. This can cause us to look in all the wrong places for what we actually already have – a tremendous sparkle, just waiting within for us to love and enjoy.

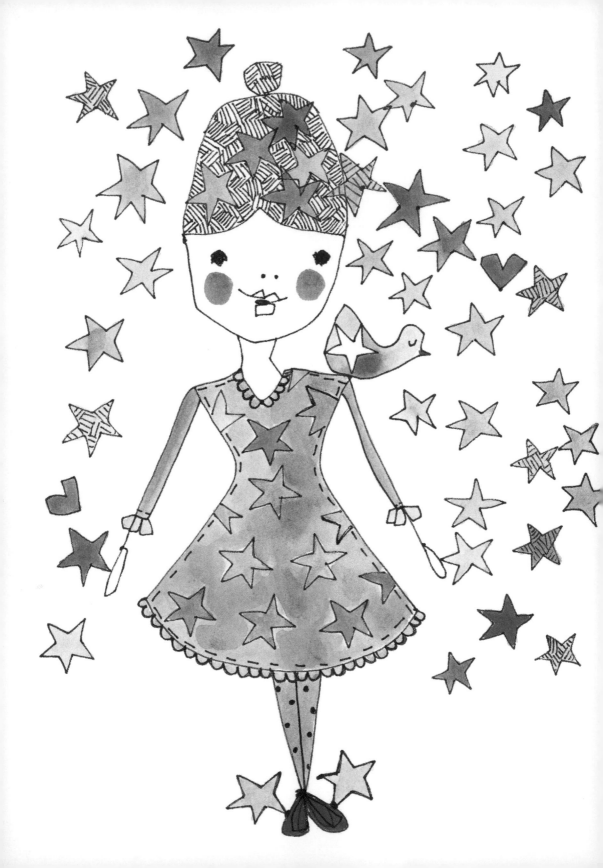

MADE OF STARS

Exploring our inner sparkle awakens us to the wonder of being alive as human beings on planet earth, amid a kaleidoscope of colour and life with all manner of creatures great and small. Indeed, we dwell in an enormous universe where shooting stars dance across the sky and moons circle planets near and far, anchored by glorious suns; in which we coexist with meteorites, black holes, galaxies, dreams, and spirits past, present and future. By astrophysical definition we are made of stars: of stardust, blown into the universe with the same Big Bang with which our universe as we know it came into being. When we acknowledge this incredible truth, we understand that we sparkle by design.

The notion of sparkling is enchanting and uplifting, conjuring images of twinkling stars and things luminous and beautiful. Just as the stars shine brightly above us, we human beings sparkle too. Indeed, each one of us possesses an unwavering, brilliant spark of life that radiates from within, a glow strengthened by our loving attention and care.

Each and every one of us is part of, not separate from, all of the magic in our universe. We human beings contain all the energy, beauty and creativity of our universe within us. We intuitively know this; we simply forget it most of the time and need to be reminded. We are miraculous gatherings of living, breathing molecules, water and energy. We are inextricably, forever linked to all life, creativity and creation. This notion may sound wild but it is the truth of who we are, biologically and spiritually. The more we connect with the magic that is within us, the more we sparkle. The more humbled and grateful we feel, the more inspired, expansive and alive we become. In my eyes, the most precious and luminous part of ourselves, our inner sparkle, is our wellspring of timeless magic and power. When we find and nourish our inner sparkle, we cannot help but lead wonderful lives.

DWELL ON
THE BEAUTY
OF LIFE. WATCH
THE STARS, AND
SEE YOURSELF
RUNNING WITH
THEM.

Marcus Aurelius

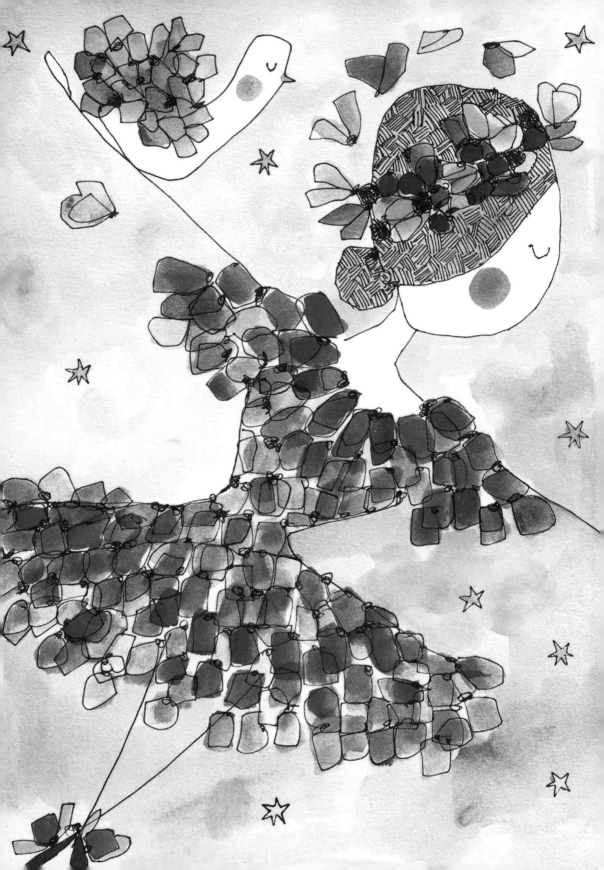

TO SPARKLE

Most of us feel overwhelmed by the grander picture of our existence,
so much so that we often deny or ignore it completely.

If our earth could speak, she would tell stories of times in which human beings lived
in harmony with the rhythms of the universe, intuitively aware of their divinity. Times in
which magic, mystery and spiritual richness reigned supreme. This tremendous historic
wisdom is part of us all.

We too infrequently acknowledge the magic that colours our daily lives. Indeed, while
all manner of miracles unfold within and around us, we limit our perspective and, as a
result, we begin to feel lacklustre. We tick boxes of to-do and already done, good and
bad, right and wrong. We expend precious energy ruminating over often unimportant,
inconsequential things at the expense of our happiness. When we live unaware of our
ever-present inner sparkle, without a sense of magic in life, we lose touch with our innate
value, creativity and magnificence.

Our spirits love to be welcomed fully into our present moments. They love to be
acknowledged, nurtured and appreciated. We are most happy, relaxed and fulfilled when
we connect, think and act from the deepest, most divine part of ourselves. Indeed,
we suddenly possess all the secrets and mysteries of the universe as our inspirations.

Acknowledging that we are derived of stardust, we begin to harness the remarkable
energy and vitality that is us. With a sense of curiosity and purpose cultivated through our
gratitude and wonder for life, we are more compelled to embrace our light and contribute
meaningfully to this world. There is a magical nexus between our self-care and collective
wellbeing on earth. When we nurture our own sparkle, we possess the energy to shine.
Not only to illuminate our own path, but as lighthouses for those with whom we share
our world.

It is important to remind ourselves every day that we are made of stars. To refresh
and re-energise our perspective. To immerse ourselves in learning about our spirits,
our earth and our cosmos. To step out of our day-to-day microcosms and forgetfulness
into a spectacularly broader, more magical picture of life.

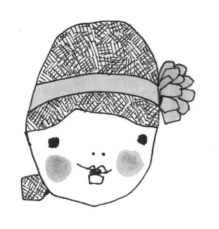

A ROSE IN
YOUR CHEEK

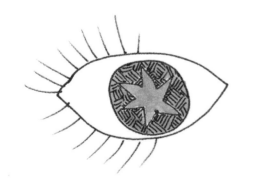

A SPRING IN
YOUR STEP

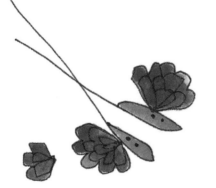

A TWINKLE
IN YOUR EYE

A SPARKLE
WITHIN

Spirit Talk

While our spirits are such vital parts of us, it seems we talk very little about them. So what are our spirits, how can we touch them, and why do they sparkle so brightly?

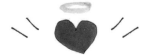

While they like to think they run the show and we often unwittingly let them, the highest essence of ourselves is not our thoughts. If we can notice, intercept and change our thoughts, we must exist beyond our thoughts. We are the thinkers of our thoughts!

What about our emotions? Are they at the helm? While our emotions are also essential parts of us and, a little like our thoughts, fancy themselves to be in charge, our emotions are not our highest essence either; they are expressions of it. Real emotions are raw, spontaneous, involuntary, sometimes even beyond our control. By nature, emotions or 'feelings' are truthful barometers of our wild and free inner states. They are the guiding whispers from the world of our spirits into our earthly realms.

While our bodies are also very important homes for us on our earthly journey, they cannot be our highest essence. There is an intelligence that is at all times directing and affecting the health, energy, motion and vitality of our physical bodies. We need only think of our heartbeats, in-breaths and out-breaths: the things our bodies just do unthinkingly, moment to moment. The involuntary little messages from our higher selves that channel through our minds and surface in our physical bodies are also wonderful to get curious about – from the fluttering heartbeats when we are in love to the butterflies in our stomachs when we feel nervous or excited. Consider the tiredness you experience when feeling blue, or the refreshment you can suddenly feel with timely inspiration. Our minds and bodies are at all times in conversation with one another, but facilitating the chatter is a higher consciousness altogether.

Fascinatingly, as our bodies grow and change through life affected by ageing, gravity and journeys of all kinds, as our thoughts and emotions shift, there is a timeless inner part of us that glistens independently of such changes. This is where we begin to recognise our spirits, and acknowledge them as the divine, magical parts of us they truly are. Our spirits are the blissful sparkles with which we are born, and the unique lights that we continue to shine beyond earthly physical reality. Indeed, we will all one day pass into spirit again, joining all those with whom we walk and share this life. We truly are magical beings, in a constant dance with all things seen and unseen.

When asked, many centenarians (people living to over one hundred years of age) are very much in touch with their inner sparkles. More often than not, our thriving elders express a progressive, cheeky and untouchable youthfulness about them, a spiritual vitality that keeps them active, robust and alive. This unique essence of us, our spirit, is a defining energy we all possess and it shapes our lives as we know them. In my eyes, our spirit, our 'inner sparkle', is the dwelling place of our consciousness. Indeed, the words 'inner sparkle', 'spirit', 'soul' and 'consciousness' appear interchangeably throughout this book, as to me they are one and the same.

It is wonderful to realise that as children we are effortlessly aware of our spirits. We are playful, expressive and freely creative. We have imaginary friends and imaginary worlds. Fairies throw tea parties at the bottom of our gardens. Colours and textures are fascinating. Words, sounds and patterns are mesmerising. Mess is delicious, and life is perfectly imperfect. While as adults it might be unrealistic to maintain certain traits or pastimes from our childhoods, it is absolutely essential that we live with a sense of magic in life; that we make it a habit to delight our senses and enliven our spirits every day. This joyous commitment to life makes for colourful, compelling and enchanting days, invigorated by spontaneity and enriched with pleasure.

Inner sparkle

Spirit

Sacred self

Creative
consciousness

Getting Metaphysical

Our inner sparkle is made of energy. Indeed, the world as we know it, seen and unseen, is made of just that – energy. We are accustomed to seeing ourselves and all things around us as solid and material, yet, when we look more closely, we are gatherings of magical energy in motion. Quantum physics has in recent times been able to illuminate and prove the presence of an incredible field of energy that can be understood as consciousness. This unseen but all-encompassing, deeply felt energy constitutes life. Studies of energy demonstrate and help us to appreciate our interconnectedness with all creation. We are living, breathing, vibrational expressions of nature existing in miraculous, moment-to-moment synergy. Indeed, while we might see ourselves as lone stars, we are in truth twinkling parts of a magnificent constellation.

C.S. Lewis once described human beings as half spirit, half animal. He explained that as spirits we belong to the eternal world but as animals, we inhabit time. Indeed, we are spirits having human experiences, constantly reconciling the journeys of our timeless timeless, divine selves within the context of our daily lives in a material world. This could be seen as a cause for tension and, indeed, some moments may be trying, however I see this reality of life on earth as a joyous cause for celebration: fodder for constant intellectual enchantment and sensory pleasure.

With awareness of our magical interconnectedness and collective consciousness, it becomes possible for us human beings to understand the immensity of our inner wisdom, power and potential. We can see how it might be possible to expand our state of awareness and transcend our earthly plane, through practices such as yoga and meditation, for instance. Indeed, human beings have delighted in such practices over time, as ways to harmonise the body, mind and spirit and experience transcendent, wondrous states of being.

This can also explain how it is possible for us to experience remarkable coincidences or moments of synchronicity. How we can connect with people telepathically across time and space. When we think about somebody in particular and suddenly, they call. When we sense we will bump into a particular person and, lo and behold, there they are. The way we can feel a profound sense of familiarity or kinship with a perfect stranger. The way we can walk into a room and gravitate towards certain people, as if magnetised. The way we can fall in true love at first sight, or experience moments of deja vu. How we could have premonitions about future events, or visions of the past. Indeed, the insights offered to us by quantum physics make it possible for us to better understand the life of our spirits on earth, to understand how we can connect with ourselves, each other and all life in profoundly enchanting, meaningful and energising ways.

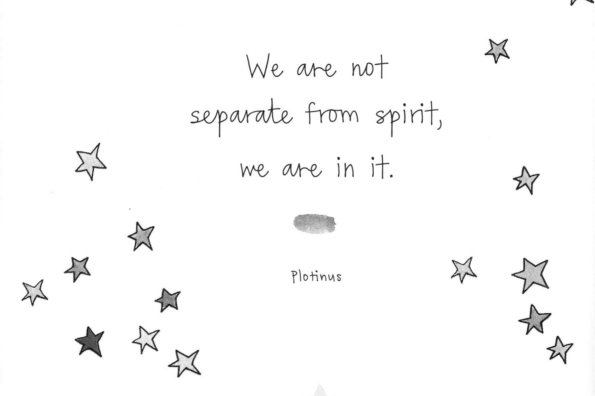

We are not
separate from spirit,
we are in it.

Plotinus

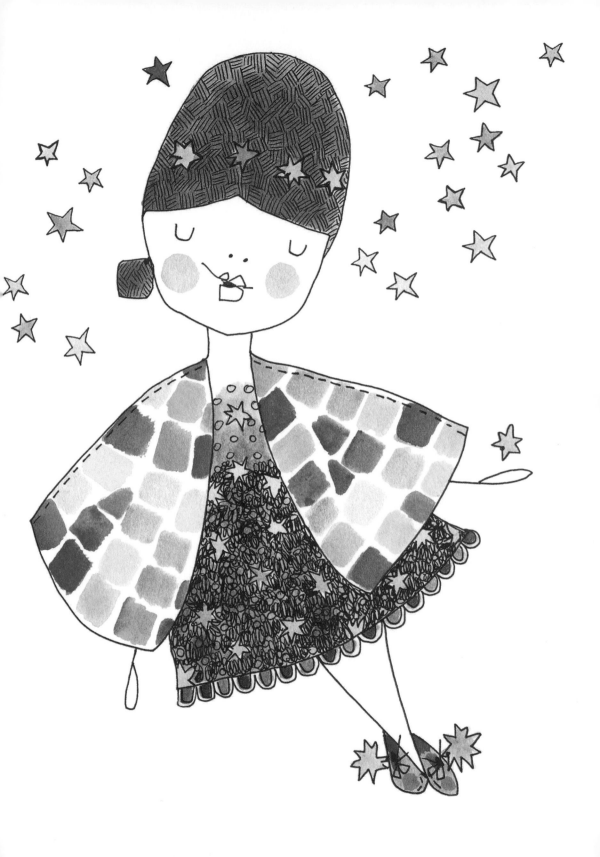

LOVE AND MAGIC

Our thoughts, emotions, words and beliefs affect us at a cellular level, shaping our wellness, radiance and vitality in profound and intriguing ways. Our minds, bodies and spirits are responsive to the environments, people, light, sound, air and other influences surrounding us moment to moment: stimuli that can either nourish or diminish our sparkles.

Unsurprisingly, this energetic reality is not exclusive to human beings. All creatures naturally sense and feel it, from our beloved household pets to animals roaming free in the wild. In recent times the emotional intelligence of plant life has also been studied in greater depth, shedding light on the phenomenally interconnected, feeling potential of all creation.

Japanese scientist Dr Masaru Emoto was recognised for his many compelling studies concerning water's response to contrasting influences. Under microscopic investigation, water that Dr Emoto had exposed to kind words, beautiful music and tenderness presented itself, once frozen, as stunningly beautiful crystal formations. Conversely, water that he had bullied, berated and bombarded with unpleasant influences crystallised into amorphous shapes. Dr Emoto captured and documented these curious findings with a series of mesmerising photographs. In further studies he noted comparisons between the crystalline water molecules of polluted water versus fresh spring water, and the spectacular transformation of crystalline water molecules blessed by a monk.

Dr Emoto's wonderful studies have since inspired many similar experiments in which two healthy pot-plants with identical exposure to water and sunlight have been subject to opposing messages of love and loathing. Studies I have sighted invariably document plants that receive positive reinforcement flourishing, and their disdained counterparts withering.

I find Dr Emoto's work provides delightful and life-affirming energetic studies celebrating the tremendous power of our love, attention and intention. It draws focus to the miraculous interconnectedness of life energy in any shape or form, encouraging us to see the sacredness of all living things and how worthy all living things are of our love. While human beings are often ready to see themselves with a great degree of self-importance, we are not superior to nature. Rather, we are interdependent, interwoven parts of her laws, rhythms and feelings of magic.

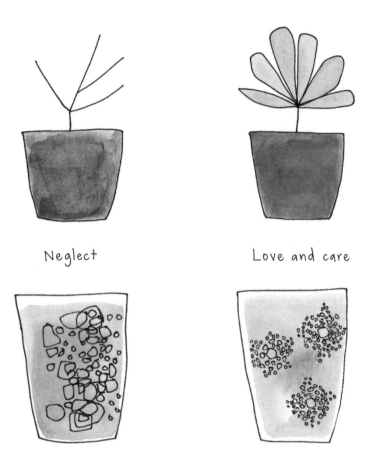

Neglect

Love and care

The tremendous power of love ♥

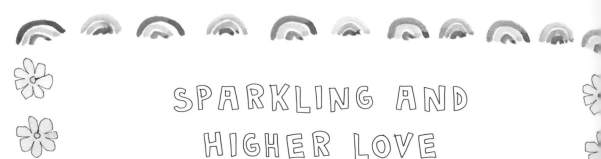

SPARKLING AND HIGHER LOVE

The spirit within each one of us is our true self and home. When we return home we connect with love. Some people call this tremendous energy Nature. Some call it The Divine or Source Energy, some name it The Universe or God. Belief in higher love has forever provided us human beings with ways to explore, honour and balance our minds, bodies and spirits.

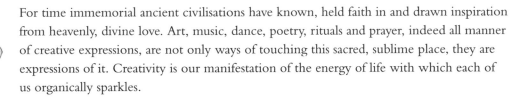

For time immemorial ancient civilisations have known, held faith in and drawn inspiration from heavenly, divine love. Art, music, dance, poetry, rituals and prayer, indeed all manner of creative expressions, are not only ways of touching this sacred, sublime place, they are expressions of it. Creativity is our manifestation of the energy of life with which each of us organically sparkles.

Through the course of time, civilisations have celebrated the energy of life in vibrant, jubilant ways. Festivals, traditions, rites of passage and rituals in honour of nature and creation are vivid examples of this luminous expression. Human cultures around the world have worshipped many different kinds of gods with riveting superpowers, some half human, half animal. Ancient Egyptian sun god Ra was often pictured in the form of a human body with the head of a falcon. It was said that Ra was born of the petals of a blue lotus, and that his tears were the source of all creation. Mesmerising portrayals of otherworldly Vedic Hindu deities such as four-headed Rudra accompany stories of the creation of the universe. In all ancient and indigenous cultures around the world sun gods, moon gods and all manner of nature gods have been cherished and revered. Worshipping nature was and will always be a way of expressing belief and gratitude in the miracle of nature. The idea of sublime energy has not only been a source of inspiration and comfort, it has drawn and continues to draw us human beings towards light and joy.

While we may worship things above and beyond our human selves, we are asked to see that sacred energy dwells unwaveringly within us. When we embrace ourselves with wonder and self-care, we feel this sublime energy moving within us. With any small act of love for ourselves, each other and our earth, we sense and nurture our divine sparkle. When we awaken to our own magic and the magic of life, we live in higher love. We craft meaningful, purposeful and deeply satisfying lives and we blossom, touched by grace and fortified by inspiration.

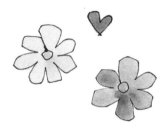

Morning Sparkle Prayer

This morning I wake up
and embrace my life –
the softness of being,
the lightness of possibility.

This morning I emerge
and float into kindness –
the loosening of fear,
the fullness of peace.

I am here,
life magically flows.

Evening Sparkle Prayer

The events of the day
have touched my mind and body.
Inside, my spirit nods gently.

The kindest, deepest
most gentle and forgiving part of me,
the stillest, most constant sparkle.

Knowing this part of me
I experience each day fully –
coming home to myself by night
in comfort and peace.

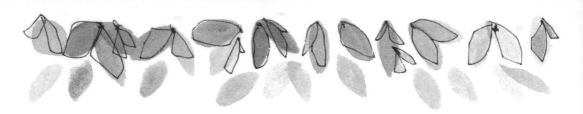

Feeling Our Sparkle

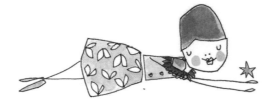

To feel our sparkle is to delight in our aliveness.

Beginning simply by noticing our breath, we can drop down from our busy thinking minds into our physical bodies. We spend so much of our lives living in the small space behind our two eyes, yet when we drop down into our bodies, and sense the flow of our breathing and the rhythm of our hearts beating, we immediately shift our awareness within and invite new discovery. Regardless of our place in physical space and time, in any moment we please we can enter our sparkling sanctuary within to retreat, relax and refresh our energy for life. In doing so, we come gently home to everything we could ever seek.

When we drop down from our minds into our bodies, following our in-breath and out-breath, we reconnect with ourselves at an entirely present, ground level. Right here and now. Most of us live in the past, pottering through our memories, or in our future, projecting ourselves into an unknown time that we are never guaranteed to have. Bringing ourselves back to our present moment via breath awareness is a humbling and awe-inspiring exercise; one that grounds and earths us while all at once filling us with divine inspiration and gratitude. With self-compassion we see that we cannot stop our minds from thinking, nor should we chastise them for being overactive. Our lives are busy and our minds think by design. We can, however, start to slow our racing thoughts, intercepting and transforming them to our advantage.

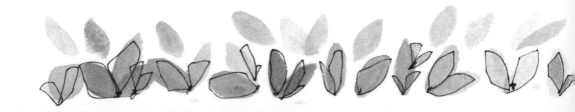

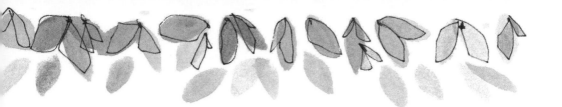

Extending from mindful breathing, we may journey to explore a myriad of ways to feel our sparkle. We can notice our sparkle glistening when we are inspired, relaxed and at peace; when we live our lives with passion and purpose; and when we care for ourselves, each other and our earth deeply. Our eyes twinkle with excitement and pleasure when we allow ourselves to be our true selves unapologetically; to be playful, creative, expressive and unique. A great way to feel our sparkles twinkling brightly is by noticing moments in which we feel happy. The exercise on page 96 is a simple but profound technique for flagging and celebrating such special moments.

Another way to feel our sparkle is by immersing ourselves in nature. Since the dawn of time human beings have been given the simple prescription to drink from nature's cup when in need of healing energy. Going into the wilderness will always be an elixir for health and happiness; a way of restoring and reviving us. We are part of nature, so coming home to nature always means coming home to ourselves.

Voltaire suggested that we are free the moment we choose to be free. In my eyes, this wisdom applies to so many states of being. I believe that we can sparkle the moment we choose to find and feel our sparkle; the moment we tune into the aliveness and vitality that is already glistening within us. In our most blissful moments, often simple and quiet moments in which we sense true gratitude for our lives, we see that real happiness isn't somewhere 'out there', it is already ours to enjoy. To realise this joy is to find and feel our inner sparkle.

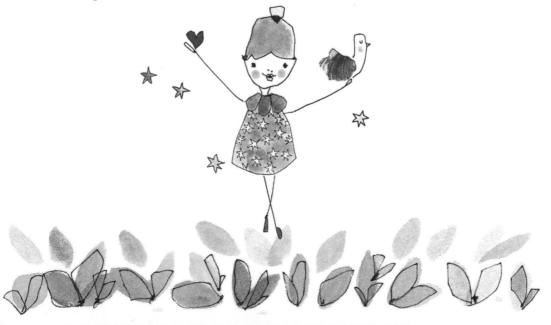

At Home Within

I always have a home.

A safe, peaceful place I can go to be myself,
to breathe and to relax,
to see myself tenderly as I am.

I simply close my eyes, breathe in and out, and there I am, at home.

I look around and see a place that I love. My heart is at perfect peace.

I feel my mind and body loosen,
and my spirit at ease.
I feel my breath begin to flow again.

At home within, the hurries and worries of the outside world melt
effortlessly away.

I am free and safe
to restore myself here in quiet bliss.
This place always was and always will be
my true home.

A place to know myself deeply,
care for myself lovingly,
and love myself truly.

Here I am now, at home within.

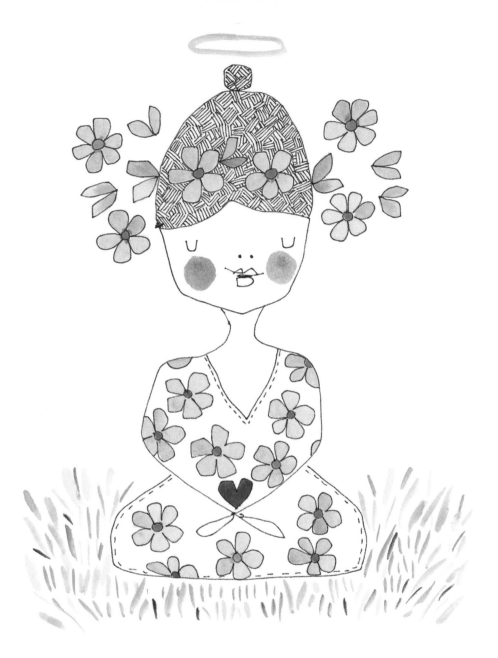

Within you, there is a stillness and
a sanctuary to which you can retreat
at any time and be yourself.

Hermann Hesse

The Joy of Sparkling

When we take the time to feel and nourish our inner sparkle we feel joy. Our days naturally become more wonder-filled, rich and meaningful. Attuning our lives to the calls of our spirits we savour the richness of our lives to the fullest, creating heavenly spaces within and around us.

We are a joy to be around when we are in touch with our inner sparkle. We are engaged, inspired and curious, and we possess a magical sense of something more. We blossom above and beyond our day-to-day jobs and accomplishments, beyond any worldly accolade or perfectly ticked off to-do list. We experience a more generous, expansive sense of time, space and potential, and emanate an effusive light and warmth to which others are drawn. Our sparkling openness makes for more joyous, connected and life-affirming experiences in daily life: experiences that blissfully reconfirm and grow the magic we feel.

In our busy world, slowing down to live mindfully and in touch with ourselves, nature and one another is a powerful, deeply healing and revolutionary act. Living truthfully with gratitude and wonder, we needn't ever feel that we are missing out on life – something we can sense when on paths incongruent with our innermost values. Indeed, sparkling joy is a sign that we are on our right path; that we are living with purpose.

When attuned to our inner sparkle, we feel energised, flexible and spontaneous. With radiant energy we can meet our daily needs on a practical level while keenly exploring the magic and mysteries of life unseen. We experience life as a wondrous, unfolding journey in which we have the power to choose our own adventure through our thoughts and actions. While experiencing the joy of sparkling might sound like an abstract notion, it is surprisingly simple. When we find our bliss within, we may find it in one another and in our world around us.

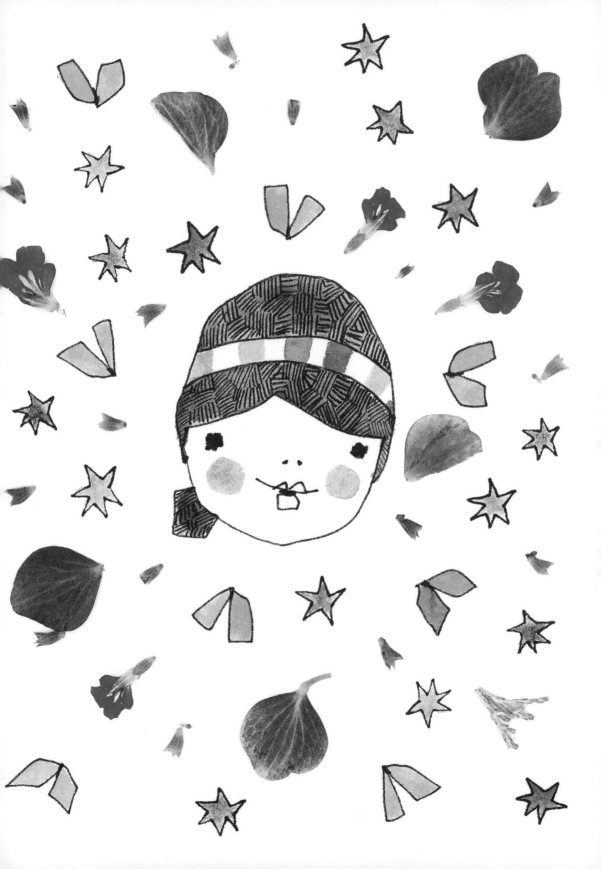

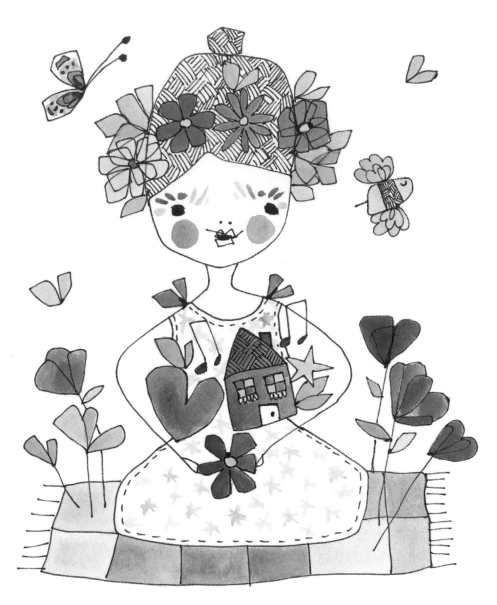

Happiness will never come to those who fail to appreciate what they already have.

Buddha

Permission to Sparkle

Giving ourselves permission to explore and share our sparkle is a gift beyond compare. We are all beings with innate creativity and integrity. We use just a fraction of our minds in daily life, connecting only just a little with our wildness and divinity. Giving ourselves permission to sparkle means connecting with the magic that we are and allowing ourselves to gracefully accept it. This might take a little getting used to, especially if we have become accustomed to dulling our sparkle.

There are many reasons why we hide our light. Perhaps we are accidentally living on autopilot, disempowered and blinded to our own magic and the magic of life. Perhaps we wish to please others by clipping our wings and staying small. Perhaps we choose not to draw attention to ourselves, dulling our sparkle because it feels like the humble thing to do. Perhaps we have become hardened or cynical to life, or feel that we aren't allowed to sparkle. Whatever our reasons may be, we must let them go. It is time to release ourselves from any old and limiting beliefs now, plant ourselves deeply into the magic of this earth and this life, and sparkle not only for our own sake but also to be lighthouses for others with whom we share our world.

We serve nobody, including ourselves, when we hide our light. We might think, 'Who am I to shine?' Yet who are we not to shine? As Marianne Williamson teaches, it is not our darkness but our light that terrifies us. We are terrified of the immensity of ourselves, our magic, our fullest, brightest potential; our oneness with everything; the grander, bigger picture of existence.

While all things in this life can be done and seen with sparkle, the hurried and agenda-driven way most of us experience life today can all too easily tarnish our vision. Without due care, our days can begin to feel like endless series of tasks that steal from our time and energy rather than renew and replenish our spirits. We can unintentionally let our busy lives diminish our radiance and limit our perspective, and find countless reasons why we can't and shouldn't sparkle. We draw on our perceived 'lack' as an excuse to hold back or deny ourselves the joy of sparkling. We cite a lack of time, a lack of energy, a lack of knowledge or some other deficit that we are permitting to stifle us.

Yet, in any moment we can see our lives as magical adventures in which we are free to choose. If each and every one of us were to sparkle, to connect with the magic of life from moment to moment, the world as we know it would radically transform. We would look, feel and act very differently. We would craft lives to nourish and elevate ourselves, soothe and inspire each other, and deeply heal our earth.

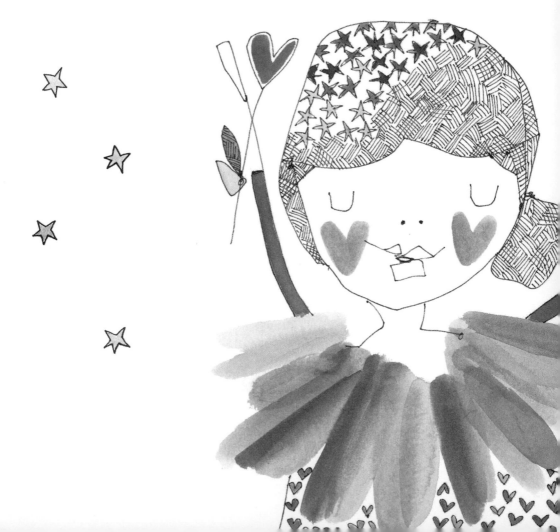

SEEING MAGICALLY

Adventure is not always about seeing new places; as Marcel Proust wrote, it is about seeing with new eyes. The moment we acknowledge that we only use such a tiny amount of our innate creativity and power, we are encouraged to think about the richness that could be available to us by expanding our state of awareness. By sharpening our wits. By opening our eyes and choosing to see with real love, curiosity and gratitude.

Wonder and appreciation are transformative companions with which we may all travel. We needn't exist on autopilot with a devastatingly limited perspective when we can broaden our faith, joy and bliss through magical thinking and living. The door is always open for us to step into a heightened, more alive state of being that is both free and precious beyond words. Living a magical life is and will always be our choice.

The experience of life holds so many joys, the best of which are unseen but deeply felt. Magical living means living attuned to the truly marvellous, sometimes subtle frequencies of life. When we explore our lives while enriched with the magical awareness of loving energy within and around us, we experience the enchanting and inspirational benefits of truly seeing. We notice precious, meaningful and guiding details, moments and opportunities we otherwise might have missed. Through our awareness of and gratitude for life, we awaken to the miraculous privilege of living.

Scientists, stoics and pragmatists past and present may view mysterious, magical states and experiences through cynical eyes. Some may dismiss the unseen world of magic, spirit, feelings and emotions as esoteric. Some disagree with the concept of a higher love, or a greater meaning to life at all. In an empirical world, we are often encouraged to see scientific, rational explanations for things. As students we are taught facts and figures and tested on our recollection and representation of data. The world of academia is based upon research that is founded on data, theories supported, proven and disproven. Surrendering to simply not knowing, or to the unknown, can feel for some like a kind of failure. Some people firmly believe that if they cannot 'see' or explain things, feelings or experiences, they cannot exist, be right or real. In my eyes, such a worldview comes at the great expense of our expansion, power and joy. I believe that to truly live, we must see magically. In my eyes, expanding our state of awareness to include the delightful mystery of the unseen world is no folly. In my eyes, opening up to seeing life magically means moving from existing in black and white to living in full colour.

Tremendous joy can become ours when we surrender our logic, suspend our disbelief and come to have deeper faith in the magic of life: the unwritten law that binds us all together. There could be nothing so freeing, humbling or healing as relinquishing our fixation with knowing and controlling things, surrendering to the divinity and mystery of things unseen but deeply felt. Seeing that we are loved, and living in an enchanting world. Seeing that life is full of wonders.

The precious, intuitive and subtle voice of our inner wisdom, the timeless knowingness of nature, speaks to us in our quiet moments of surrender. In these moments we touch the complete richness of all that is seen and unseen in this life, knowing that we are protected, loved and guided. Seeing through loving and wondrous eyes is a wholly free and revolutionary act.

The mountains and hills
will burst into song before you,
and all the trees of the field
will clap their hands.

Isaiah

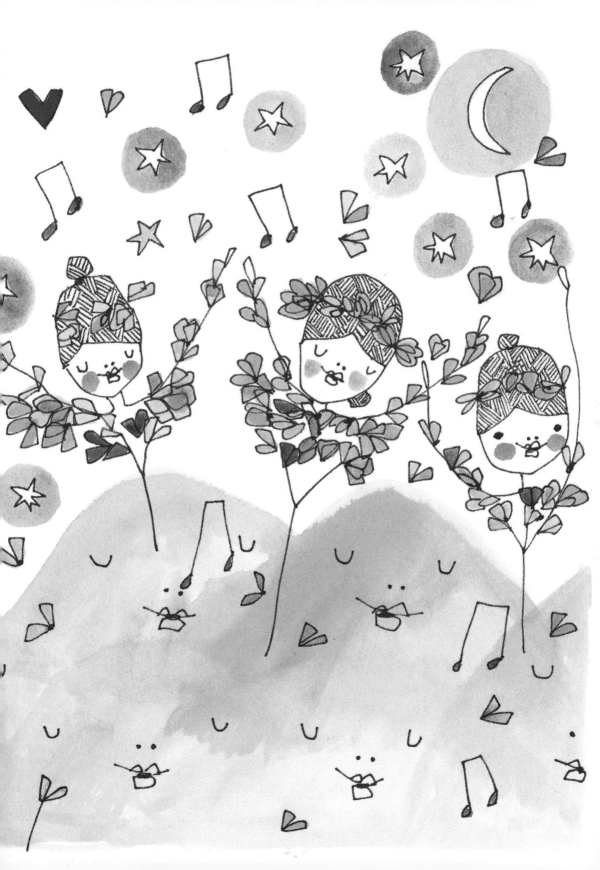

A TRAVELLER'S PRAYER

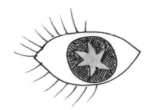

I choose to see anew today.

Things my eyes have begun to overlook

will become interesting to me again.

Details I have started to miss

will spring forward to delight me.

Moments of magic I have been passing by

will start to enchant and inspire me.

I choose to see like a traveller today,

traversing new land,

exploring new sights.

With the energy, curiosity and gratitude of a traveller

I will explore and savour all the details of my life.

I will allow my senses to be delighted.

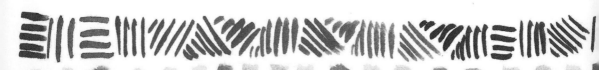

I will take in the scents, the sounds and the sights,

the colours, the shadows and the light.

I will revel in various patterns, tastes and textures.

I will notice faces, movement and touch.

Today I will notice the many magical messages meant especially for me.

I will know that the people, creatures,

words or songs that cross my path

were all meant to be met with my awareness.

I will allow my life to tell me stories,

to inspire and nourish me,

and to guide me on my way.

Today I will awaken to my life.

I will raise my head and lift my eyes.

I will refresh my spirit with each step I take,

knowing that my life is as rich and bountiful as I make it.

Knowing that gifts great and small

tickle me for my attention in every moment.

Today I choose to have magical eyes,

and to experience my world anew.

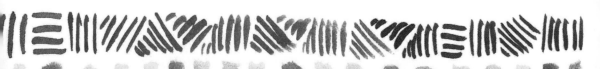

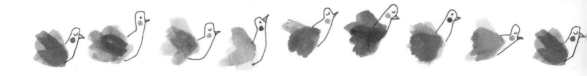

BELIEVING IS SEEING

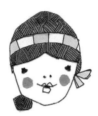

It is unquestionable that this world of ours is a magnificent place full of sublime mysteries, profound pleasures and delightful secrets, just waiting for our wits and senses to sharpen! Amid the busyness and distraction of this time and place on earth, our free spirits are calling us to embrace things unseen but deeply felt as a way of returning to our innate magic and the magic of life.

It can be said that seeing is believing, but it is equally true that believing is seeing. The more we believe in the magic, beauty and delight of the universe, the more we will see and experience it around us. The more we believe in the kindness and goodness of others, the more we will see the kindness and goodness in others. The more we believe that we live in a magical and generous universe in which we are unconditionally held and loved – in which coincidences, synchronicities, signs and symbols abound, guiding us each step of the way – the more enchanting, meaningful and fulfilling our lives become.

In infinite ways, life calls us to look more closely at things. Synchronicities, connections, messages and signs that we are meant to notice wait patiently for our acknowledgement every day. When we slow and quieten ourselves as often as possible, we begin to sense the humming magic and effortless perfection in all things. We feel our place and sense our belonging here. We notice our oneness with the tremendous energy of nature, each other and all life. We experience the fullness of our feelings, know sensory pleasures of all kinds,

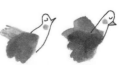

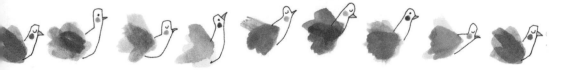

become attuned to our rhythms and the rhythms of our earth, and grow more deeply in love. While our unseeing selves suffer, disconnected and far from home, our seeing selves cannot help but experience deep joy, abundance, inspiration and peace.

In times gone by and in different cultures and places around our earth, 'knowingness' has been our natural state of being. Spirituality was organic, celebrated and central to human life. Healers existed in communities of all kinds, treating the whole person – body, mind and spirit. Natural remedies from the earth, such as herbs, flowers, pigments, scents and stones, were balms for strength and restoration. Signs found in dreams and in the stars were seen to offer meaningful guidance. Rituals coloured life, bringing a sense of togetherness and sacredness to daily experience. Human beings lived in awe-inspired congruence with the moods, seasons and wisdom of the natural world.

Our collective focus seems to have shifted away from the delicate frequencies and magic of life and onto the solidity, value, function and appearance of things. All the while, felt and mostly unseen energy within and around us constitutes and shapes our lives moment to moment. It is time for us to suspend our disbelief, awaken to magic, and dive fully into the lusciousness of life.

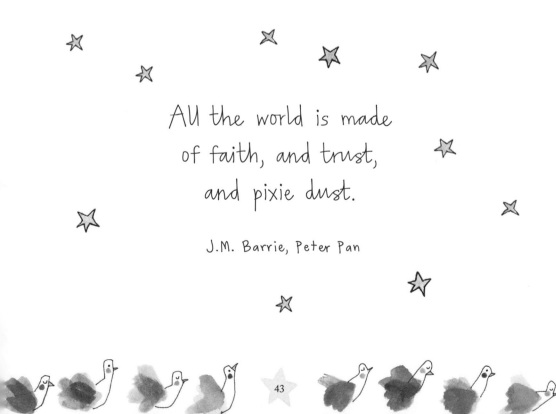

All the world is made
of faith, and trust,
and pixie dust.

J.M. Barrie, Peter Pan

Creativity and Magic

Creativity is our spirit energy. It is not reserved for artists, poets and writers; it is a gift each one of us possesses. We are innately creative beings, and inspiration is all around us.

When we are inspired we are 'in spirit', touched by divine influence. A history of inspiration has resulted in innovation, art, beauty, music and literature from which we draw profound inspiration today. The work we do now will leave a legacy for those to follow us, and it is our responsibility to leave this world a better place through our own loving, creative acts and visions.

Perfectionism, self-criticism and 'growing up' at the expense of our playfulness are just some of the forces that stifle our innate sparkle. Educator Maria Montessori wrote that 'Our care of the child should be governed, not by the desire to make him learn things, but by the endeavour always to see burning within him that light which is called intelligence.' Indeed, the learning and exploration we pursue throughout our lives should continue to ignite the light within us and delight our spirits.

We are all inclined towards different forms of expression. Writing, drawing, cooking, inventing, knitting, singing, crafting, gardening, song or poetry writing, sculpture, dancing, collage, woodwork and countless other creative, sensory pleasures await our exploration. We can all be moved by nature, words, art and music, and by expanding our vision through experiences, travel and exploration. When we come to know other human beings we connect, and our creativity expands its potential all the more. Indeed, being creative together can result in tremendous, transformative collaborations far exceeding our expectations or our solo efforts. Our perspective can widen to encompass fresh ideas as we merge our own imagination with the thoughts and ideas of others. Exciting new directions cannot help but emerge when we come together in creative spirit.

Immersed in creative endeavours, we dip into flow states that, like meditation, expand our awareness and awaken our spirits. Inviting more delightful moments of creative bliss and flow into all our days is a sure way to awaken our inner worlds. Indeed, the more we explore our creativity, the more we sparkle.

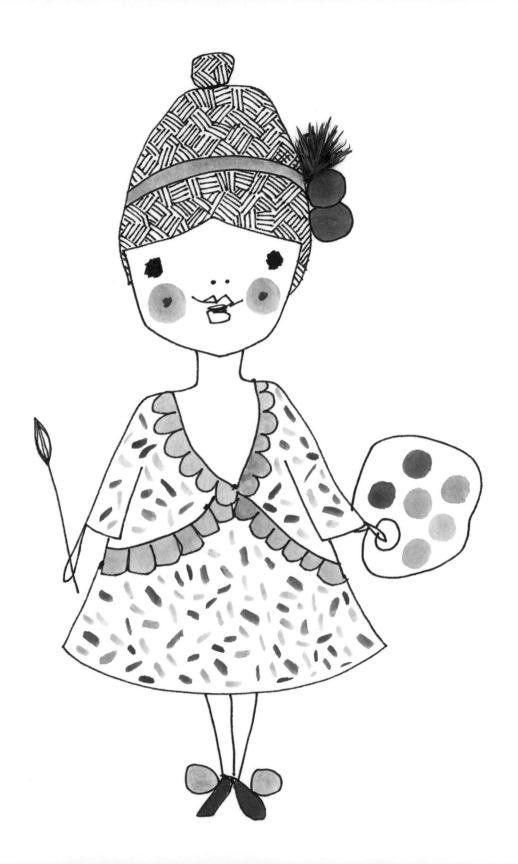

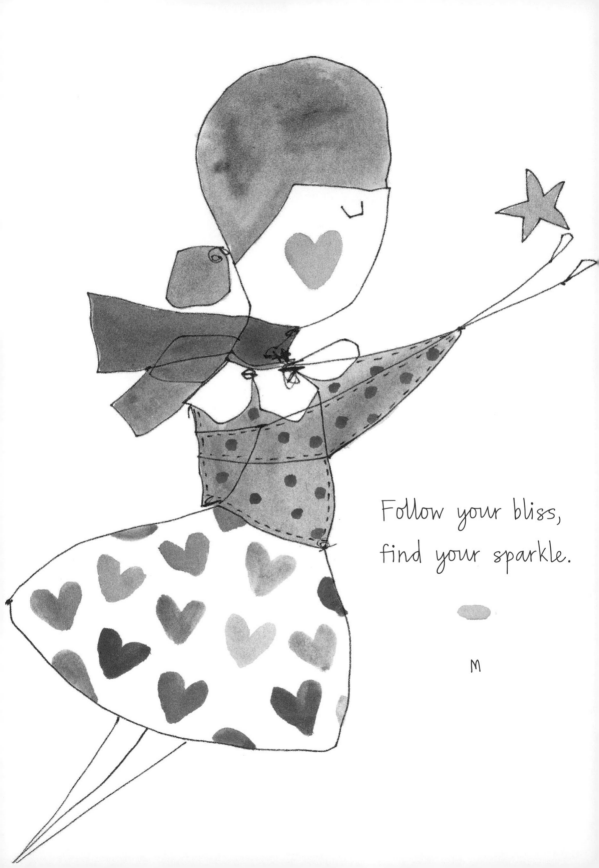

Follow your bliss,
find your sparkle.

OUR BLISS AND PURPOSE

In choosing what to do with our time and our lives, we are wise to chase our bliss and pursue the things that ignite our spirits. Indeed, exploring our inner sparkle is a wonderful way to realise our purpose and calling in life.

It has been said that if we love what we do, we need never work a day in our lives. It is not selfish – it is in fact extremely important that we follow our bliss. In doing so, we are able to make a real difference in this world with our passion, creativity and expression, whatever it is that we are doing. We might be making art or teaching children, building or growing things, perhaps caring for others. In any case, following our bliss with effort and integrity, it is natural that the material aspects of our lives will be divinely looked after for us. That we will never be short of riches, nor wanting of anything. While this sort of magical thinking might take an enormous and courageous leap of faith, in my eyes, I have only ever seen purpose-driven living rewarded beyond measure.

All that we require when actively seeking our purpose is an openness to experiencing joy and bliss. Rumi wrote that 'Everyone has been made for some particular work, and the desire for that work has been put in every heart.' By following our bliss and activating our passion, we allow the energy of our sparkle to carry us, in flow, through life. We are encouraged to see that life can and must indeed be fun, and that we can and must enjoy ourselves unapologetically, freely and fully. Even in the face of our greatest challenges, the chance always exists for us to find and grow our bliss.

This lighter, freer and more spacious take on life breaks free from old models in which our gains were seen as the result of our pains and struggles. Let's embrace the notion that gains can be made through choosing joy. Through less pushing and more softening. Less striving, more ease and grace. That we can arrive at the finishing lines of our greatest dreams not breathless and overwrought but sparkling with our fresh inspiration to go forward.

Let self-acceptance
free your spirit.

Approve of yourself,
and sparkle from
within.

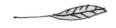

M

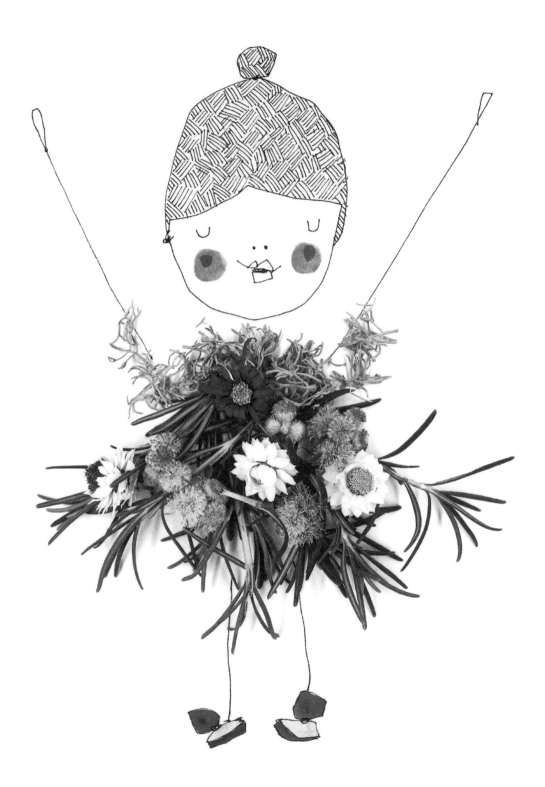

AIMING HIGHER

Today I aim higher.
Like a beautiful flower in bloom,
my petals reaching up into the sky,
I see myself blossoming too.

I allow myself to merge into
higher energy now:
to feel the feelings I wish to feel,
to see myself the way I wish to see myself.
To know myself in the way I wish to know myself,
and to gift myself my own approval,
for which I so deeply yearn.

No matter where I am right now in this very moment,
I know that my spirit is free.
My spirit is sparkling.

Breathing on I sense myself blossoming effortlessly.
I grant myself permission to rise now
like a flower towards the sky,
knowing that I am ready to grow.

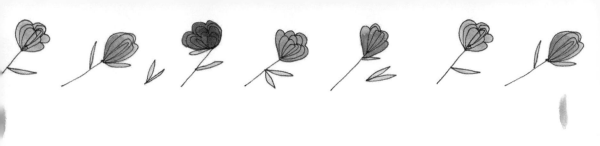

As I blossom I see myself happy, healthy and fulfilled.
I see myself radiant, confident and at peace.
In elevating my vision, I elevate my spirit now.
The beauty I can see within and around me,
I create.

I capture a clear vision of my most radiant self,
and I keep this picture firmly and safely within.
In this picture I am flourishing, joyous and alive.

I know I may merge into
this graceful vision of myself at any moment,
gathering magical courage and energy
with which to rise up, sparkle and shine.

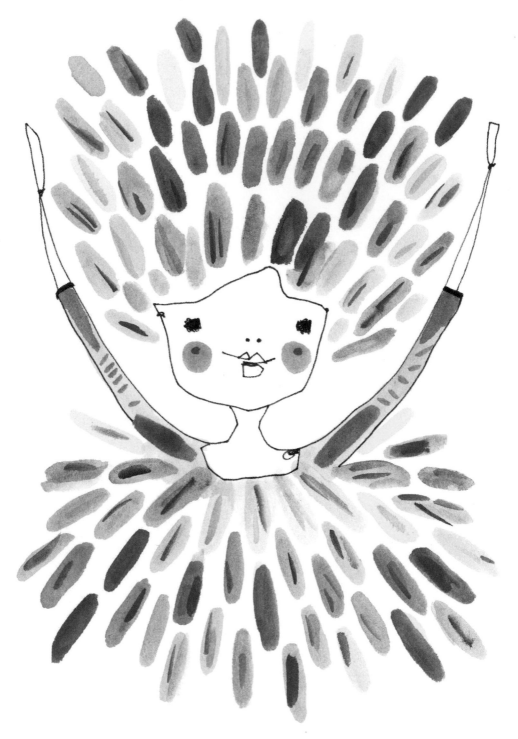

Creativity is intelligence having fun.

Einstein

SPARKLING, YOUR WAY

It is true that we sparkle just by being alive. Indeed, the unique spirit
with which we came into this world is our glittering life force: our own
original inner glow. Rather than lose ourselves in comparison with others,
we need to polish our own unique sparkle.

We often see others as brighter, better and more beautiful than we are. This is partly
due to the fact that we are often blind to our own magnificence, but it is just as much
a symptom of the culture of comparison in which we live: a culture we have normalised
at our own very great expense.

Comparison of ourselves with others is a gateway to unhappiness. It can unnecessarily
ruffle our sense of self-confidence and self-worth, cause us to overlook our own unique
beauty and potential, and thieve our joy. To combat this, we can catch ourselves in the act
of comparing ourselves to others and affirm ourselves by saying, 'I am me, and this is my
life.' We can appreciate the attributes and offerings of others while remembering the truth:
that we are all divine, worthy and complete, just as we are.

Observing our culture of comparison we realise that constantly measuring ourselves
against others is not only futile, it is making us deeply unsettled. We can never walk a day
in someone else's shoes, nor are we meant to. What other people do is their creativity,
their expression, not ours. We are here to respect, support and learn from one another,
not to compete and compare with one another. We are here to live unique, authentic
and joyous lives – to enjoy and honour our sparkle and to allow others to do the same.

When we truly see ourselves in each other, touch even for a single moment upon our
shared humanity, the senselessness of our competition and comparison with one another
becomes palpable. By nurturing respect and appreciation for ourselves and each other,
we can move forward together in true creativity and peace.

No one's sparkle should dull our own, nor should our radiance dull others' light. When we stop comparing and uplift one another instead, choosing to take joy in each other's joy and actively celebrating each other, we set ourselves and one another free at last. As Rumi reminds us, we are born with wings. Why do we prefer to crawl through life? Indeed, we were not born to struggle and suffer. We are here to be loving, creative human beings. The lifelong pleasure of sparkling is found in setting ourselves free to love, enjoy and affirm our lives and ourselves, moment to moment. There could be no greater gift than this, nor a more wonderfully satisfying way to live.

DO NOT GO WHERE
THE PATH MAY LEAD,
GO INSTEAD WHERE
THERE IS NO PATH
AND LEAVE A TRAIL.

Ralph Waldo Emerson

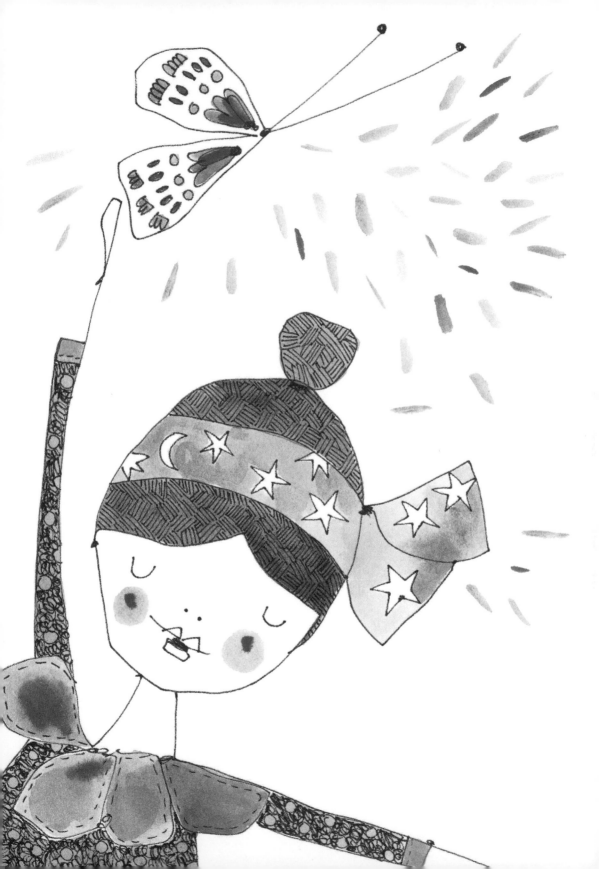

THE SPARKLE OF INTUITIVE WISDOM

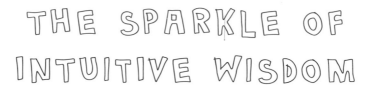

There are so many things in life we simply cannot know or control. Surrendering to not knowing and relinquishing our need to control all parts of ourselves and our lives is in fact tremendously courageous and powerful. Indeed, surrendering opens up more space for more magic to blossom.

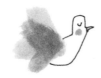

Embracing the unknown, mysterious and spontaneous parts of our lives with wonder awakens us to precious inspiration and guidance. When we surrender to not knowing things we are encouraged to go within, feel our feelings and connect with our intuitive wisdom. Deep beneath our overthinking, stress and fear, we find the ever-present peace and quiet that exists within us. In this peaceful spaciousness we can receive the precious intuitive messages awaiting us.

Sometimes we need to lose ourselves in order to find ourselves again. Sometimes by listening to our inner sparkle we can suddenly find ourselves catapulted into unplanned and life-shaping journeys that our spirits truly desire. With humility and openness, and by allowing divine grace and intelligence to guide us, magical adventures become ours to enjoy.

Profound knowingness sparkles within us in every moment. Indeed, within each one of us dwells infinite intuitive wisdom to which we have unlimited, lifelong access. By connecting with our intuition, our inner wisdom, we may gracefully navigate all the moments of our lives. Sometimes we are simply too loud or busy to hear the whispers from within. Sometimes we are too distracted seeking others' advice or approval. Maybe we are just too busy controlling and ordering everything. The secret to accessing our inner wisdom is to surrender gracefully, quieten down and listen in.

When we expend a lot of our energy busily controlling, perfecting and planning all aspects of our lives we can find that the deliciousness of spontaneity and other unexpected pleasures of life can elude us. We allow no room for pottering, no space for our imaginations to float free. No opportunity for life to reveal the enchantment and spaciousness we seek. In this way, surrendering makes us more open, humble and flexible human beings. Our conscious surrendering lets life in to work divine magic in ways we could never possibly script.

Unburdening ourselves from the need to know and control all things frees up precious energy with which to sparkle on, enjoy ourselves more fully, and chart wonderful new territory in life.

Happiness, not in another
place but this place . . .
not for another hour,
but this hour.

Walt Whitman

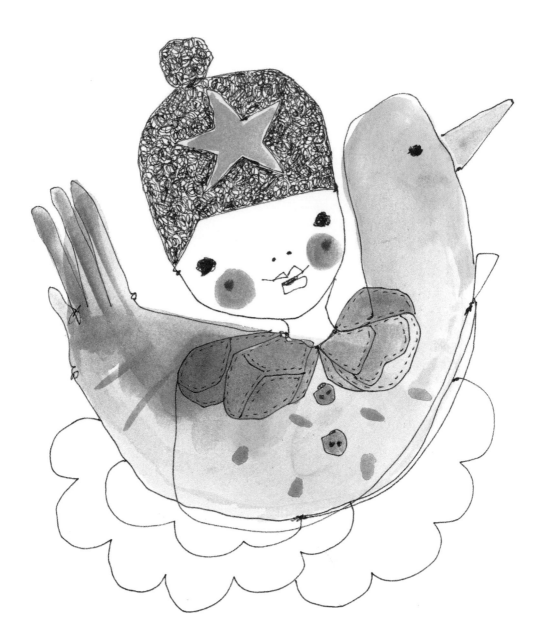

Don't be satisfied with stories,
how things have gone with others.
Unfold your own myth.

Rumi

WRITING YOUR OWN STORY

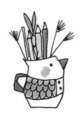

At any moment, we may step outside the illusion of 'normal' living to design and enjoy our own lives with greater flexibility and innovation. Certain things are unavoidable or necessary in this life, but the rest is much more fluid and flexible than it appears. Indeed, our lives are up to us. Reclaiming free and creative thinking and intelligently, consciously subverting the status quo can lead to great adventure, not to mention immense contentment.

Making changes to live a more unique, authentic and magical life in alignment with our innermost values might be very appealing, yet for some there seems to be no inroad in sight. We might feel stuck in circumstances we have created or accepted. We might feel weary of spirit, and see little potential for personal transformation. Maybe we worry that there might not be a safety net ready to catch us when we start to shift spaces or feel things more deeply. When we traverse new ground far deeper and more expansive than we could ever have imagined, we might wonder if the people with whom we share our world will still love and approve of us if we change our lives . . . As Margaret Shepard reminds us, sometimes all we have available to us in order to move forward is a courageous, wholehearted leap of faith.

Unfulfilled desires of our spirits can manifest as sadness, fatigue, restlessness, regret, ill health and other undesirable states of being. When we courageously tune in to a more expansive sense of our true personal freedom, approving of ourselves first and foremost without the need for all others to validate and agree with us, we may chart new territory for ourselves, recharge our energy, and fall back in love with ourselves and life. In living bravely and authentically, we also pave the way for others to explore the potential of their creativity and dreams.

It is encouraging to know that it is our human nature to be drawn to the light. As Arthur Eddington wrote in his book *The Nature of the Physical World*, 'Whether in the intellectual pursuits of science or in the mystical pursuits of the spirit, the light beckons ahead, and the purpose surging in our nature responds.' Indeed, when we heed the calls of our inner sparkle, we are ushered into the light. When we bravely take steps ahead, we begin. We needn't see the whole staircase and know exactly how we'll climb it – we just need to take the first step!

At all times, we should honour ourselves as co-creators of our own deeply rewarding and soulful journeys. When we have a big dream that emanates from our spirit, we do ourselves a great service to fully explore all possibilities and not be discouraged by others' aspersions or disapproval. Indeed, in the words of Albert Einstein, 'Great spirits have always encountered violent opposition from mediocre minds'! Go forth, sparkling.

FAITH IS TAKING
THE FIRST STEP EVEN
WHEN YOU DON'T SEE
THE WHOLE STAIRCASE.

Martin Luther King Jnr

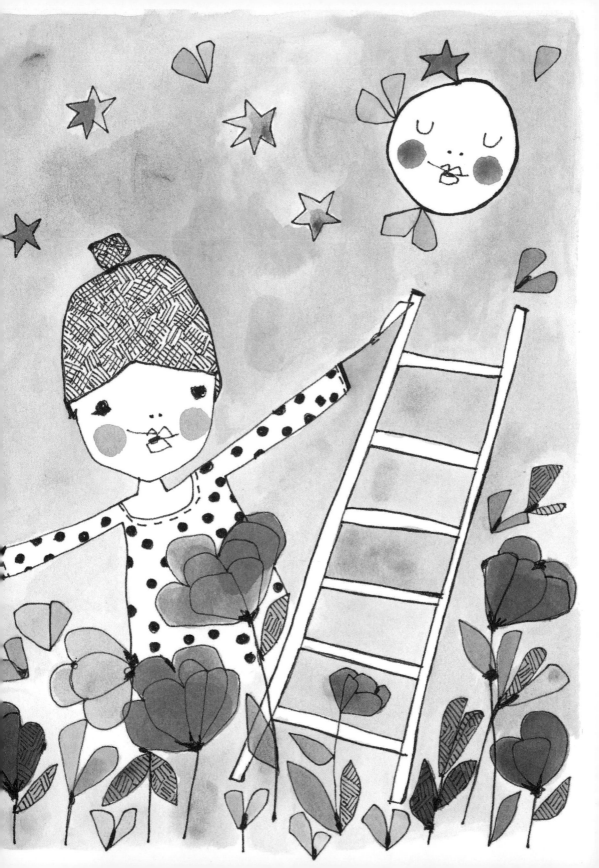

GREAT SPIRITS
HAVE ALWAYS
ENCOUNTERED
VIOLENT OPPOSITION
FROM MEDIOCRE
MINDS.

Albert Einstein

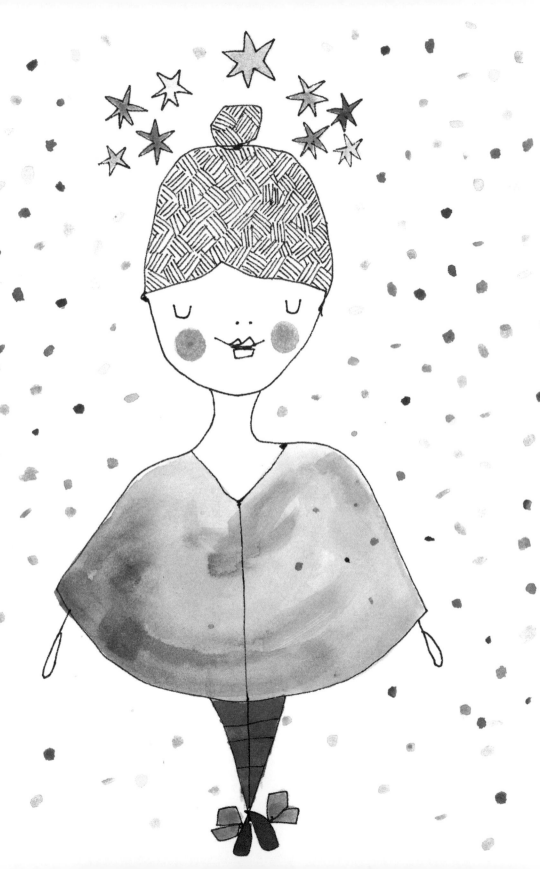

Sparkling Meditation

I take a moment to close my eyes and relax now.
I inhale deeply,
pause for a moment at the very top of my breath,
then exhale fully out, soothing my whole body.

Breathing deeply in and out again,
I visualise letting go of any loose thoughts,
hurries or worries. I let them fall away.
This is my moment to quieten my mind, right now.

I have nothing more, nothing less to do.

I imagine a little sparkle at my heart's centre.
Like the first star to appear at dusk,
this little sparkle twinkles gently but surely within my heart.

With each breath in and out,
I visualise this twinkling star growing a little brighter,
and a little brighter again.
Breathing in and out, breath by breath,
filling my heart with sparkling light.

As I breathe on, I imagine the light of my sparkle
emanating from my heart and moving through
my entire body now, illuminating everything.
I take my time visualising sparkling light circulating
within me, touching any areas of my body
that need special love and attention in this moment.
I feel my whole body sparkling as I breathe on.

When I feel ready,
I allow the light of my sparkle
to circulate beyond my body,
creating a field of energy around me
in which I may move through the world.
I sense the air around me
tingling with my own magic.
Breath upon breath, moment to moment.

Checking in again with my little star now, I bring my attention
back to my heart centre. I draw the tremendous light and energy
I have cultivated back, deeply, firmly within me now,
securing it with each breath, back to my heart.

Inhaling and exhaling gently on, I feel my sparkle.

Journal Prompts

To me, my sparkle is . . .

I felt my sparkle within or around me when . . .

If there were no rules or expectations I would . . .

If magic was assisting me moment to moment, I would ask it to . . .

I feel most in touch with my sparkle when . . .

I would like to be admired for . . .

To me, generosity of spirit means . . .

The aspects of my spirit that I admire are . . .

The things that are keeping me from sparkling are . . .

I might be able to move through by . . .

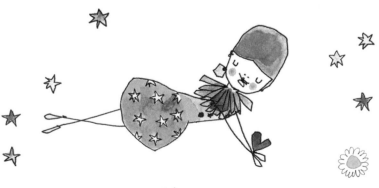

Affirmations

MY SPIRIT IS SPARKLING

I AM FREE TO BE MYSELF

I LET LOVE LIGHT MY WAY

I SEE THROUGH GRATEFUL EYES

I LET GO AND LISTEN IN

MAGIC DANCES WITHIN ME

I AM NEVER ALONE

I TAKE GREAT LEAPS OF FAITH

MY COURAGE GROWS EVERY DAY

MY SPIRIT IS FREE

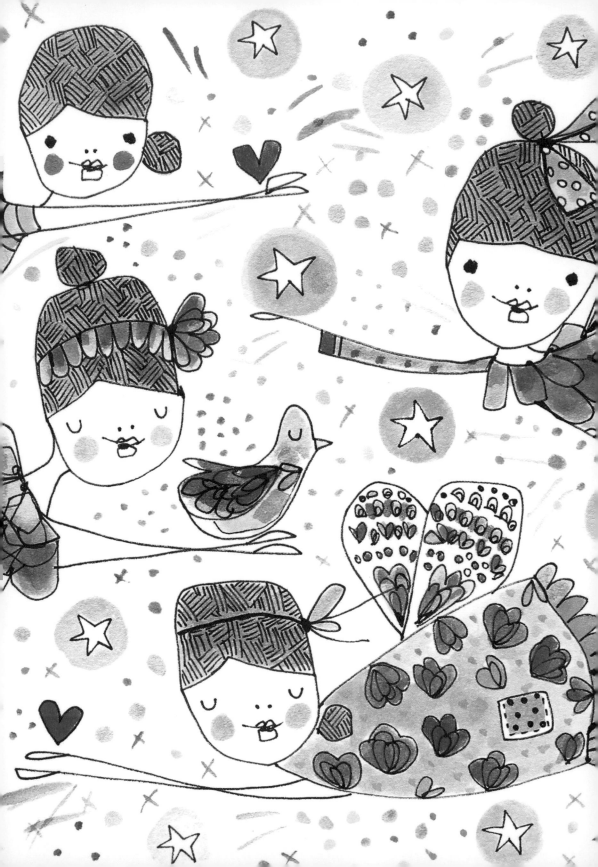

NURTURING
YOUR SPARKLE

Nurturing our spirits is often the missing piece in our collective quest for happiness, fulfilment and radiant health. Our world desperately needs our love, and we are called to be at the helm of positive transformation by cultivating kindness, compassion, courage and creativity within ourselves.

We are capable of so much more than we know. Thinking and seeing magically is possible for each and every one of us, opening up a whole new world of possibilities and expanding our awareness of the tremendous energy within and around us. Explore your own healing powers, see happiness as a virtue, choose in favour of your bliss, and settle into a deep, purposeful and fulfilling sense of belonging in this life.

This section is brimming with practical approaches to nurturing your spirit in daily life, with actionable thoughts and ideas ready to support, uplift and inspire you.

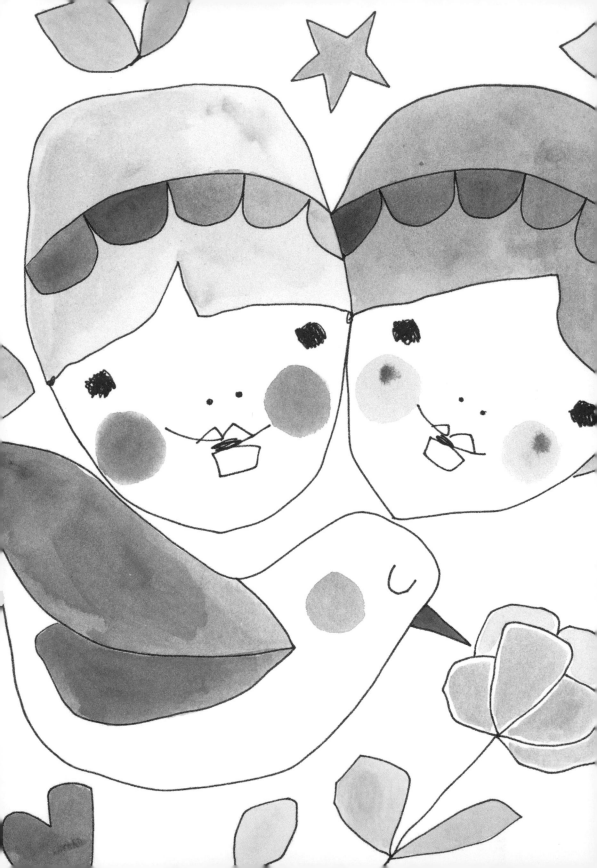

Magical Living, Modern Life

Many of us can feel depleted in the face of busy modern life in a material world. Perhaps we push on day to day, over-filling our schedules and feeling far too busy to rest, relax and care for ourselves. Perhaps we are anxious and not sleeping well. Perhaps we are striving very hard towards a particular goal and our balance of work, rest and play feels right off kilter. Whatever the case may be, re-establishing connection with our spirits is an empowering way of embracing ourselves and our lives with healing, energising love.

In what has been an age of consumption and distraction, we are beginning to see that our connection to ourselves is of utmost preciousness. The grace we come to embody through deep self-awareness and care allows us to be authentic and present in all the moments we live.

In order to live fulsome, magical lives in our modern world we are being called to notice and integrate the different layers of our sensory experiences. We are being invited to acknowledge the multidimensionality of our humanness, and tend lovingly to the worlds both within and around us.

Danish philosopher Søren Kierkegaard expressed it beautifully when he described human beings as syntheses of the infinite and finite, temporal and eternal, freedom and necessity. Indeed, delighting, comforting and expressing our timeless free spirits in the context of a physical world of day-to-day responsibilities, activities and relationships is a conscious form of art. When we take the time to listen lovingly to the calls of our spirits and embrace the magic all around us, we cultivate truly fulfilling lives.

Buddha says that if our compassion does not include ourselves, it is incomplete. Indeed, caring for our minds, bodies and spirits with loving compassion and tenderness is not selfish or indulgent; it is simply essential. When we support ourselves to truly enjoy our lives, we sparkle from deep within. We possess energy with which to be kind towards others, to explore our dreams, and to contribute meaningfully while here on earth.

SPARKLING BASICS,
HERE AND NOW

We can nurture our sparkle in so many delightful and satisfying ways: through the thoughts we think, the actions we take, and the noursihing foods we choose to eat.

Our thoughts are choices that we make, moment to moment, and they shape our actions and experiences. Regardless of how we might have thought up until this moment, magical thinking is available to each and every one of us, right now. Awareness of our present moment is mindfulness, and mindfulness is essential to our personal and collective sparkling on earth. Buddha reminds us that what we do today matters most. We must know that it is truly possible for us to embrace ourselves and the magic of life, right now.

Just as we have chosen so many things in our lives, we can choose to think kinder, more patient and generous thoughts and, in doing so, become kinder, more patient and giving human beings. We can choose to nurture our spiritual wellness by championing joy, wonder and playfulness, and by practising gratitude rather than taking things for granted. We can choose compassionate listening and full presence over quick judgement and distraction. We can choose to support, uplift and inspire one another rather than compare and compete with each other. Positive thoughts empower us to act in ways that bring real joy to ourselves and others.

Like our thoughts, our words are made of energy and possess great power. If we wish to sparkle, we must speak in ways that elevate and inspire ourselves and those with whom we share our world. Our words can be hurtful or healing, limiting or radically empowering. Try this now. Think or say the words 'I can't . . . ', 'I don't . . . ', 'I shouldn't . . . ', 'If only . . . ', 'I'm too busy . . . ', 'Tomorrow . . . '. Ugly. Terrible. Awful. Pause.

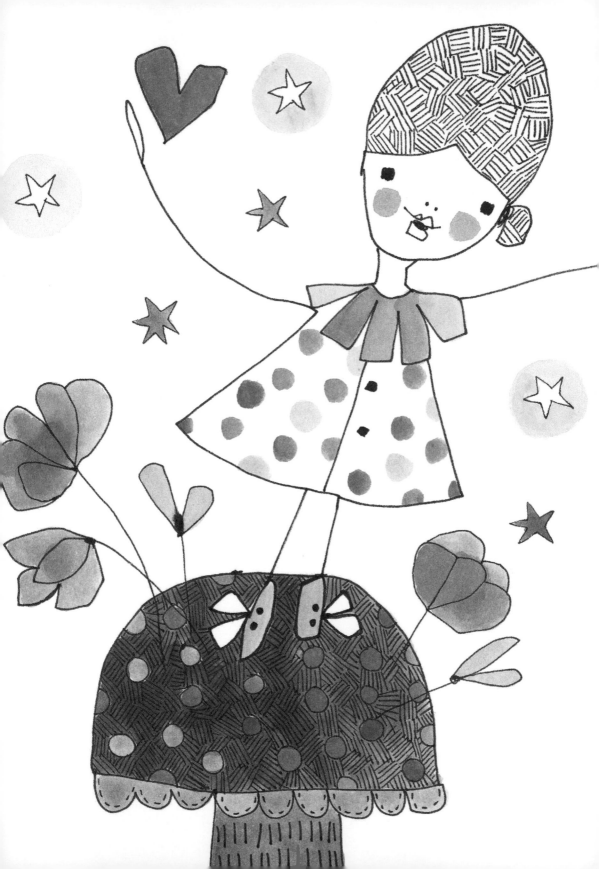

Can you feel the low vibration of these words dulling your sparkle? Now feel into these words: 'I can . . . ', 'I do . . . ', 'What if . . . ', 'I have time for that! . . . ', 'Today . . . '. Beautiful. Wonderful. Brilliant. Can you feel the difference? When we come to see that everything is pure energy, including our thoughts and words, we awaken to our own tremendous power. By choosing high-vibrational, uplifting thoughts and words we can sustain a positive mindset for life, express ourselves with passion, live our lives to the fullest, and foster more nourishing relationships with ourselves and each other.

We can all too easily forget that our everyday actions become our life stories. Indeed, practising kindness, gratitude and compassion, exploring our creativity and doing things we love in ways we love with people we love are all ways to sparkle. Learning new things, changing scenery, exploring our earth, looking up at the stars, taking a different path and, indeed, choosing to see the 'pixie dust' in our daily lives are all ways we can refresh our spirits. It is exciting to realise that the many actions that can nourish our sparkle are undeniably joyous, life affirming and, more often than not, absolutely free. We are called to look at the actions we take in all our relationships, in the work we choose to pursue, and in the ways we choose to rest, relax and move our bodies. The thoughtful actions we take enable us to lead truly nourishing and meaningful lives.

The way we move our bodies is an expression of our sparkle. The body language with which we communicate including our gestures, posture and the way we move through space indicates how we feel inside and expresses the way we see the world. Crossing our arms, hunching our shoulders and keeping our heads and eyes cast down are just some examples of body language that can diminish our sparkle. Just as choosing written or spoken language to nurture our spirits in daily life, choosing positive body language and carrying ourselves gracefully can go a great way towards sparkling. Simply putting our shoulders back and lifting our heads can be transformative and empowering, from one moment to the next. Try it now! Our minds, bodies and spirits are in constant conversation. Connecting the energy of our inner sparkle with our physical bodies is fortifying, healing magic.

As far as action goes, let's get physical! Moving our bodies helps to clear and refresh our minds, energise and strengthen us physically and mentally, and recharge our spirits. Sometimes feeling lacklustre is a call to move our bodies. Movement creates fresh energy, allowing our vibrance to return to us. A brisk walk or a quick swim, a set of stretches or breaking into spontaneous dance can very simply and swiftly reinstate our sparkle. When our bodies are stagnant, our minds and spirits can follow. Sometimes we just need to get moving physically in order to get upwardly mobile on every level.

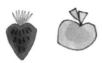

While it's easy to forget, the food we eat becomes us: our organs, bones and blood. Our physical bodies renew themselves completely many times over the course of our lifetimes, and to sparkle in mind, body and spirit we are wise to build ourselves on high-vibrational fresh and whole foods. Natural approaches to body care also nurture our sparkle – what we put onto our skin is absorbed into our bloodstreams and is worthy of our thoughtful care.

Nurturing our inner sparkle is a pleasure and, with our commitment, becomes a lifestyle we want to pursue. When we consciously follow and nurture our sparkle, we naturally feel more relaxed, buoyant and energised. Feeling lighter and more joyous, it follows that we experience the freedom and vitality for which we inherently yearn. When we ignite and nourish our spirits our happiness, self-worth and resilience blossom. We feel compelled to make positive and supportive decisions for ourselves, and allow ourselves to enjoy our lives to the fullest, at last.

SING LIKE NO ONE
IS LISTENING.

LOVE LIKE YOU'VE
NEVER BEEN HURT.

DANCE LIKE
NOBODY'S WATCHING,

AND LIVE LIKE IT'S
HEAVEN ON EARTH.

Mark Twain

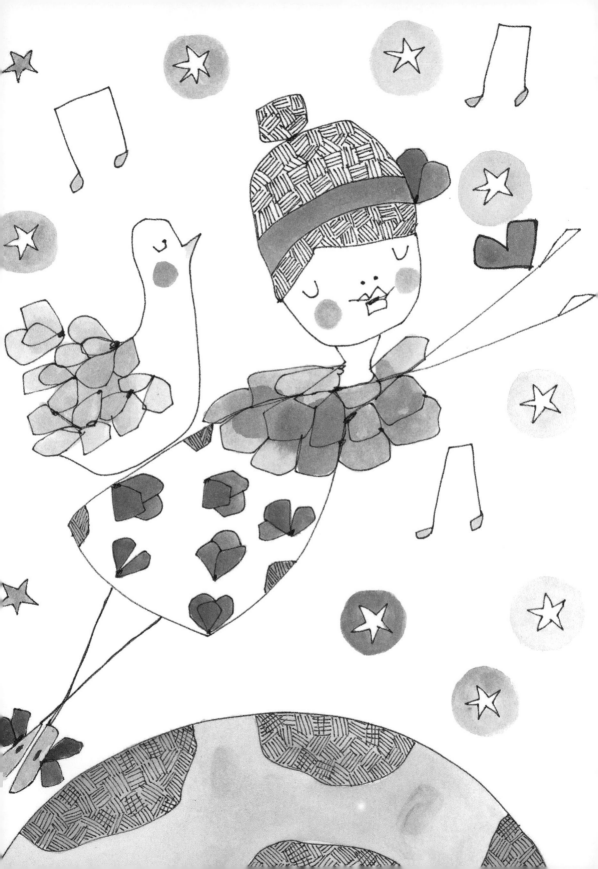

Spirit Wellness

Caring for our spirits is an essential part of cultivating radiant wellbeing in daily life. While we hear a great deal about various diets and exercise regimes as ways to achieve the sparkling wellness we seek, we are also being invited to shift our thoughts, actions and language around wellbeing now. We are being called to partake in higher conversations around kindness and gratitude, joy and inspiration, stillness and grace: spiritual arts that elevate and fortify us from the inside out.

While we might do all we can to design lives in support of our health and happiness – very important things such as eating well, exercising, keeping our homes neat and clean, cultivating good manners, and the list goes on – when we forget to connect with and care for our spirits we will always sense that something very important is missing in our lives. We will feel a niggling imbalance or incompleteness in all our moments and days.

In the stressful rhythms and pressing circumstances in which so many of us now live, it is no wonder that our inner sparkle can feel a little lacklustre. We often race from one activity to another, eat foods that are disconnected from nature, and perform kinds of exercise that can stress our bodies rather than fortify and nourish them. Constant stress in daily life deeply affects not only our sense of inner peace and balance, it also affects all the cells, organs and workings of our bodies, making it difficult to sparkle. It compromises the energy within us, and shapes the energy we emanate. The pandemic of ill health we are experiencing now has devastatingly direct links back to chronic stress.

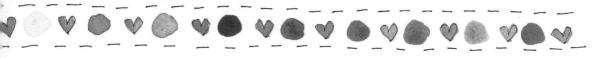

Many of us isolate stress to a mental experience – something that is happening in our minds – all too often forgetting that our bodies and spirits feel with us too, moment to moment. Certain stresses, such as nervous excitement or tension under the acute pressure of a challenging life experience or impending deadline, are normal sensations of aliveness. Many of us have begun to exist in a state of hurried automatic pilot, though, a state in which we are oblivious to the amount of stress we are truly feeling and the toll that it is taking on all aspects of our being. Stress affects everything: our bodies, minds and spirits, thoughts and actions, our relationships, moods, perspective and clarity.

It naturally becomes harder to see and embrace the magic of being alive when we are depleted at the spirit level. We can eat kale for breakfast, lunch and dinner but if we are stressed, ungrateful, unkind and ungenerous, we will not find the sparkling wellness that we seek. We can exercise to a perfect, personalised program week to week yet if we aren't present in our present moments, feel perpetually anxious or are endlessly critical of ourselves and others, we will feel weak and exhausted. We can get eight hours of deep sleep a night but if we ignore opportunities to be of loving, meaningful service to others in our waking lives we will feel imbalanced. We might go on adventures but be so distracted en route that we miss all the magic around us. We might then wonder why we feel dull or empty, for it is in giving that we receive, and in noticing that we see.

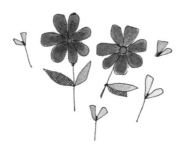

Our wellbeing is essential to our enjoyment of life on earth, not to mention the health and happiness of those with whom we share our lives. We can, and are entitled to, savour our lives to the fullest, feeling sparkly, fulfilled and complete. The key to sparkling wellness is attending to our spirits honestly and respectfully, without judgement or fear. We are often quick to notice our shortcomings and perceived flaws before acknowledging the immensity of our strengths and achievements: the courage, perseverance and generosity of our spirits. Truly knowing and caring for ourselves means connecting with the fullness, richness and depth of our complete humanity. Loving and caring for our spirits in the way they deserve is real nourishment.

DELIGHTING OUR SENSES

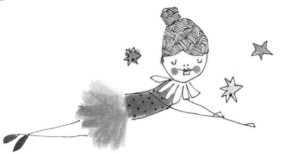

When we delight our senses, we awaken our spirits. Think of the tenderness and connection of touch, the inspiration and enchantment of music, the sublime deliciousness of real food, the freedom and ecstasy of movement, the gravitas of beautiful words, the dreamy colours in a rainbow, or the bliss and peace of unhurried, mindful walks amongst nature. Indeed, when we are mindful and grateful on our paths each day, we can feel our spirits brimming with fresh energy and aliveness.

Choosing joy every day is a simple but truly transformative way of nurturing our spirits. Committing to smiling and laughing more is a gift for our sparkle, even if such a practice feels unnatural to begin with! On average, children smile over two hundred times a day – while grown-ups are apparently hard pressed to smile just twenty times. Smiling relaxes all the muscles in our faces that can become terribly tense, and sends signals to our brains that we can relax. That all is well.

Laughing, especially belly laughing, is so enriching that it is used therapeutically to reduce stress and anxiety while boosting mood, immunity and vitality. Laughter therapy sessions, which participants attend simply to laugh raucously together, happen worldwide week to week. In the 1970s American journalist Norman Cousins famously attributed laughter to relieving himself of the debilitating symptoms of chronic illness. He watched back-to-back comedies, discovering laughter as an effective form of pain relief. Becoming fascinated with the biochemistry of human emotions, he went on to write articles identifying and exploring human emotions as keys to our sickness and health. In my eyes, this is subject matter well worth our further investigation! Smiling and laughing are sparkle-nurturing techniques that take instantaneous effect and are free for all of us to explore.

Rituals are also very nurturing and grounding for our spirits in daily life. We are by nature creatures of habit and we love being in rhythm. It might be a visit to your local cafe to order your usual favourite. It might be taking up the same table at your favourite restaurant. It might be writing in your diary upon waking or tucking into bed at night, recording your dreams, thoughts and ideas or the events of the day. It might be cuddling your pet or kissing your beloved before saying goodnight. It might be taking a certain walk with a friend or family member each week, savouring movement with meaningful conversation. Whatever rituals you thoughtfully create in your daily life, allow them to nourish your spirit with delight, comfort and joy.

There are so many simple and daily ways to nurture our inner sparkle. Making time to rest and relax, taking time to breathe, or practising affirmations and visualisations to soothe and energise ourselves are wonderful remedies for our spirits. Giving ourselves permission to mix good doses of fun into the more routine aspects of our daily lives is an effective and pleasurable approach to expanding our joy. Living attuned to the gifts of our senses – what we see, touch, hear, smell and taste in the world around us moment to moment – invites great pleasure and inspiration, allowing us to feel our inner sparkle and returning us to the magic and potential of now.

As a result of nurturing our spirits we feel brighter about ourselves and life. We naturally boost our immune systems, elevate our moods, care for the health of our hearts, touch all our cells with the healing powers of love, and become happier, healthier people. There is no positive act too small or simple when it comes to nurturing our spirits and embracing the magic of our lives. We can begin with one grateful thought a day. One smile. One prayer. One random act of kindness. One deep breath. In this very way, we begin to sparkle.

A SPARKLE-NURTURING LIST FOR YOU TO GROW...

Spending time with loved ones

Spending time alone

Having soulful conversations

Walking in nature

Laughing

Smiling

Singing

Dancing

Cuddling

Diving into the ocean

Looking up at the stars

Practising affirmations

Enjoying self-care rituals

Watching the sun rise and set

Pottering through autumn leaves

Nestling into a warm bed when weary

Waking up to sunshine

Being kind towards others

Being kind towards ourselves

Listening to beautiful music

Learning new things

Slowing down

Taking breaks

Changing scenery

Practising yoga

Exploring creativity

Exploring mindfulness

Breathing deeply

Being curious

Being playful

Decluttering

Choosing real, whole foods

Choosing natural beauty care

Noticing our own gorgeousness

Believing in a magical universe

Believing in ourselves

• • • • • • • •

• • • • • • • •

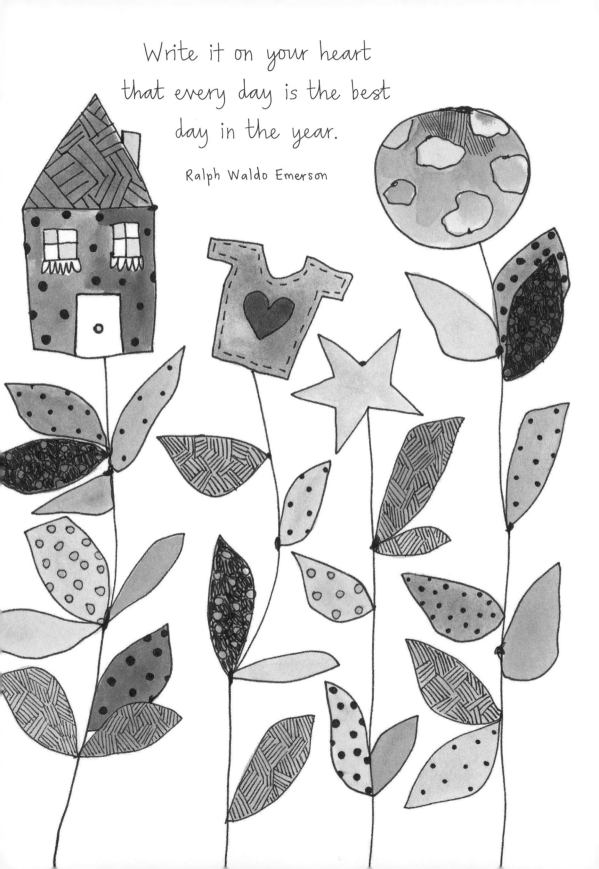

Write it on your heart
that every day is the best
day in the year.

Ralph Waldo Emerson

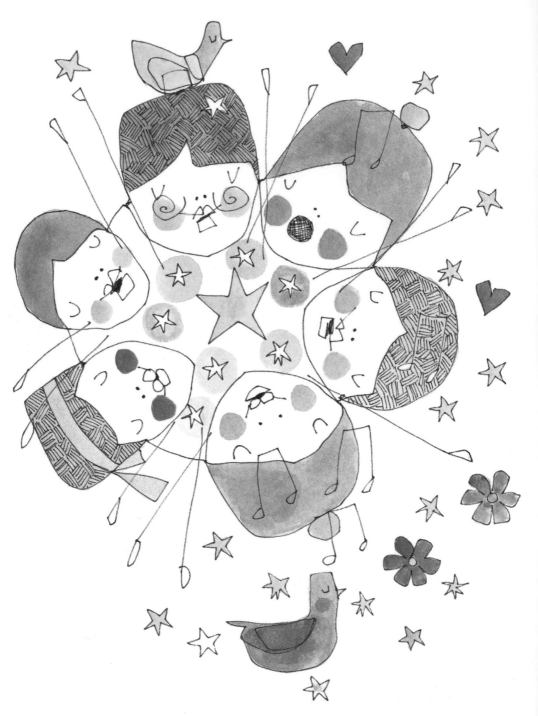

There is nothing in the world so irresistibly
contagious as laughter and good humour.

Charles Dickens

INSTANT SPARKLE FIXES!

Even when pressed for time or feeling uninspired, there are simple things
we can do in our daily lives to reignite and polish our sparkles.

Might wearing a special hat put you in a good mood? Might singing or listening to a great podcast make your work or travel all the more light and breezy? Might you take the time to visit a farmers' market to connect with your community, starting your weekend right and filling the heart of your home with nourishing produce?

Might you choose to stay in bed that little bit longer on a weekend, snuggling in with a book, your loved ones or your pets, just to nurture that very important part of you that needs quietness and tenderness? Might you take that moment longer to help someone else, to listen to them or offer them a helping hand? Practising kindness and generosity are powerful ways to keep our sparkles radiant.

Might you enjoy a luscious walk in nature or find an accountability buddy to enliven your exercise routine? When we actually enjoy the movement we choose to do rather than see it as a chore or, worse still, a form of punishment, we bring so much more joy to our minds and bodies. Might you actively declutter your diary, leaving breathing room for whims, downtime or adventure? Making time and space for spontaneity, freedom and pleasure are guaranteed sparkle fixes.

Why not plan a little getaway or organise a dinner party, and for extra fun, inspire your guests with a theme for dress-ups? Bring out some board games for all the more giggles. Good old-fashioned fun, from piñatas to pin the tail on the donkey, never fails to bring people together! Get messy out in nature, with some paint, or in the kitchen. Just let go. Be imperfect. Make some waves.

One of the tragedies of life is that we feel we need to become serious as we 'grow up'. Keep a sparkle in your eye, be young at heart and choose to have fun. Call on instant sparkle fixes whenever you need a boost, and you'll be sure to create a truly magical life.

SPACIOUSNESS AND SPARKLING

As we awaken to the true richness of our lives, we realise that, contrary to what has become popular belief, more doesn't always mean more. Filling every waking hour with commitments can leave us feeling stressed and strained, while quiet time, rest and relaxation revive our sparkles. Overfilling our minds and environments can leave us feeling cluttered and overburdened. On the other hand, consciously slowing down our racing thoughts, paring back our busy schedules and decluttering the spaces around us allows our spirits to float free.

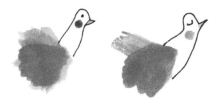

We are and have always been enough. No extra bells or whistles are necessary for us to sparkle – no extra things, accolades or trimmings. Our current consumer culture encourages us to believe that the next best trend, thing or feather in our cap will make us sparkle, suggesting to us every day through advertising and media of all kinds that we are missing or lacking something – that we need more to grow our happiness. Alas, we're disillusioned when we feel the same after the temporary shine has worn off our new shoes, our new car, diet plan or gadget. We see such things do not make us happy – and if they do, it is only until we secure the next thing we covet. Fleeting satisfaction like this can understandably leave us feeling unsettled, wanting and incomplete.

Believing that we are not happy, balanced or beautiful enough is a story that serves our pulsating global economy while simultaneously creating much of our daily stress and anxiety. Every year we spend more money on cosmetics cars, clothes and coffees . . .

the list is endless. If we were to simply acknowledge the truth of our human strength and beauty, to connect with ourselves, each other and life in deeper, richer and more meaningful ways, we would save unthinkable amounts of time, energy, money and angst.

More money can buy more things but more things don't seem to be bringing us more happiness. The concept of spiritual bankruptcy speaks to the idea that we can become poor and empty inside, our inner worlds deficient or completely ignored, despite the riches that might colour our outer worlds. Indeed, the more things we have in our lives and on our agendas, the less time we actually have for ourselves. By striving for happiness through accolades, things or others' approval we can find ourselves compromising our true selves to 'succeed' in life, in our own or others' eyes, or to make things work. It is no surprise that chasing worldly gains at the expense of our spiritual richness leaves us stressed, strained and profoundly compromised. If we were to see that living mindfully with gratitude and generosity of spirit brought us true happiness, so much competition, comparison, clutter and disappointment could be circumvented.

Feeling constantly hurried and out of touch with the rhythms of our earth deeply affects our vitality, equanimity and spaciousness. Many of us work indoors, wake up hurried and rush out the door, leaving no time to enjoy the sunrise, stargazing, earthing or pottering around: simple things that have healed, restored and replenished human beings over immeasurable moons. All things said and done, we are part of nature and need to heed her ways. Mother Nature takes her time and achieves all that she needs without hurrying. As Ovid reminds us, a rested crop makes for a beautiful harvest. There is a season, a rhythm, a time and a place for everything. Energising sunrises follow dark, restful nights; vibrant rainbows follow clouds and rain; little buds blossom into magnificent flowers. We are crafted of the same intelligence as all living forms within nature. We need only to respect, love and learn from the wisdom of nature to gain precious, healing insights into our own lives.

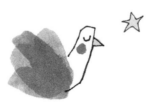

We are very quick to say that we are very busy and have no time. We even compare our busy agendas and bustling lives. When we slow down, however, we can do things well and with love. Living slowly, time miraculously expands to accommodate us and suddenly we do not feel time-poor, we feel time-rich. Through our mindfulness we create greater spaciousness in and around ourselves, and our lives flow in a far more efficient, entirely different way. By embracing the joyous magic and richness that life can bring, our experience of time radically transforms. Our days become less like hurried races to mobile finishing lines and more like decadent, deeply rewarding journeys.

Sparkling happiness is not somewhere 'out there'. It is not another person, place or thing. It has been inside and around us all along. Such a revolution in our spirited thinking needn't mean that we become listless or unmotivated people; quite the contrary. In my eyes, by slowing down and supporting ourselves to flourish from deep within, we will finally find the vital energy and balance for which we have been yearning. Debunking the idea that our things or our productivity equate to our self-worth or success allows us to enjoy ourselves, just as we are. We can literally be more by having and doing less.

Spaciousness and lightness can be cultivated through mindfulness exercises that quieten the mind. Taking time to enjoy visualisations, meditations and gentle yoga practices that combine movement with breath awareness are wonderful examples. Decluttering our spaces helps to circumvent overwhelm and breathes light and air into our lives. Actively retreating and quietening down to enjoy downtime allows us to listen in to the calls of our spirits and recharge our batteries. Indeed, sometimes there is nothing quite as luxurious as a walk outside, an early night and a little bit of time alone. A homemade card and a tender embrace can be more of a gift than any extravagant or expensive present ever could be. A picnic prepared with love and enjoyed amongst nature can feel more indulgent than silver-service fine dining at a fancy restaurant. Great joy can be found in simplicity and spaciousness, and in appreciating the wisdom that less can be so much more.

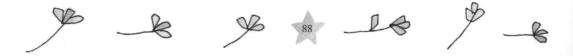

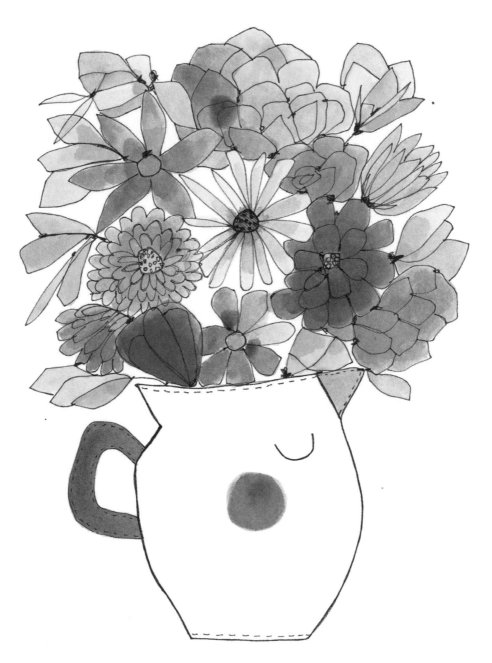

Nature does not hurry,
yet everything is accomplished.

Lao Tzu

To see a world in a grain of sand and a heaven in a wild flower, hold infinity in the palm of your hand and eternity in an hour.

William Blake

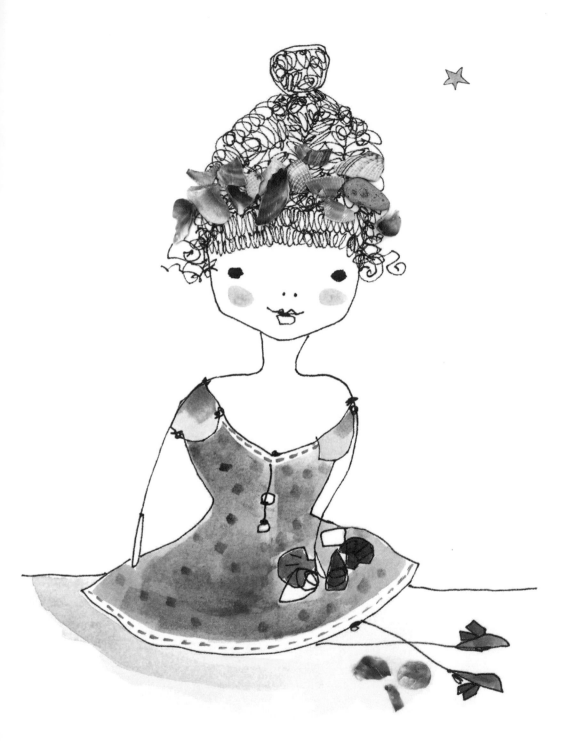

MAKING TIME EXERCISE

Time poverty has become something we almost compete over. We are always somehow busy, very busy, or busier than ever before! Many people wish to make positive changes in their lives, incorporating yoga, dance or daily meditation, for example, but claim that they simply have 'no time' at all. The truth is, we all have time: the same twenty-four hours in any given day. The point of difference is our priorities: what we choose to value the most, the things we 'make' time for, not 'find' time to do.

I once heard Louise Hay describing her relationship with time. She suggested that when she needed more time she would mentally 'stretch' it with the power of her thinking. Conversely, when she wanted time to pass more quickly for whatever reason, she would use the power of thought to compress it. She suggested that time was flexible and that we could all practise this fun technique, making time work for us, rather than against us. I agree with Louise. With time on our side we can certainly embrace the fullness, richness and beauty of our lives with peace and joy. While the notion of time being elastic might sound terribly esoteric to some, quantum physicists would suggest that it is completely possible as, like all things, time is what we make it.

On the next occasion you find yourself saying that you have 'no time' for things you truly want or need to do, catch yourself. Check in with your priorities and see how you could better structure them in support of your happiness. Talk gently to time, asking it to expand so that you can achieve all the good things you wish to on any given day. Ask time to love and support you in every way.

Rather than saying or believing that there's never enough time, try to correct yourself by thinking and saying, 'There is always more than enough time for the things I want and need to do.' Celebrate time, and make each moment count. Indeed, time can pass us by when we are distracted and mentally absent in our present moments. Simply returning ourselves to where we are, right here, right now, is a way of expanding, honouring and enjoying time.

Let time become something luxurious and abundant in your life. Begin with your thoughts, turn your thoughts into speech, and follow your words with affirmative actions. Proactively transform your relationship with time, and find your sparkle deeply nourished.

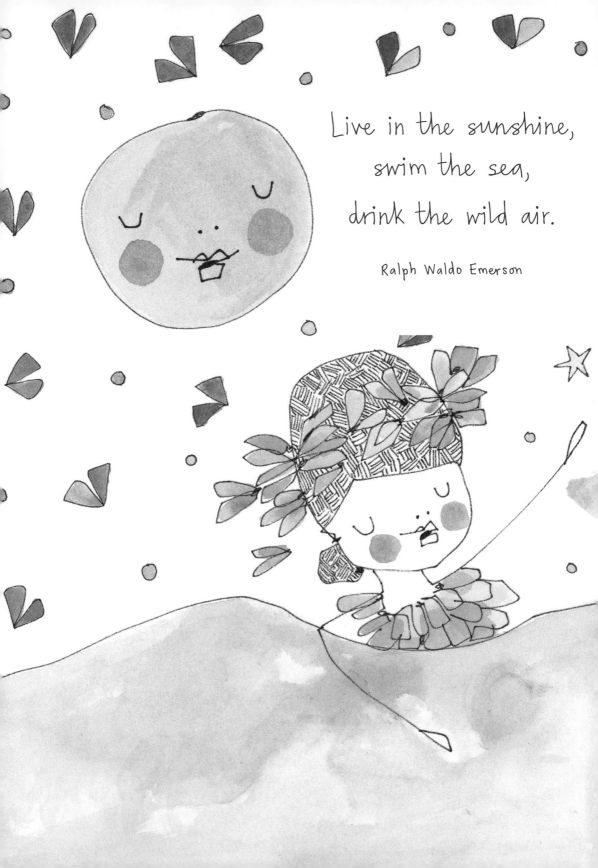

Live in the sunshine,
swim the sea,
drink the wild air.

Ralph Waldo Emerson

ONE THING, ALL THINGS

We sparkle with the same glow as all creation. In living joyous
and mindful lives we are called to see God, or The Universe, in all things.
In the Japanese Shinto religion, Kami are seen as gods that dwell in
all things, even inanimate objects such as vases or life forms such as
fruit and vegetables. In this way, all things we touch need to be
treated as special and sacred.

The gratitude and care we give to our personal belongings, our home environments,
the ingredients with which we cook and indeed anything in our lives that we touch with
our minds, hearts and hands is a joyous and profound way of showing our respect for the
magic in all things. We are often brusque, careless and forgetful with our possessions, even
to the point of accruing clutter that complicates and burdens our lives. Yet when we touch
things we love, it naturally follows that we need less things in our lives to be happy. What
we do have simply matters more. Acknowledgement, love and appreciation for all things,
big and small, changes our lives. In the words of Socrates, the secret to happiness is not
found in seeking more, but in developing the capacity to enjoy less.

Buddhist philosophy suggests that the way we bring our mindful attention to one thing
is the way we bring it to all things. For example, kicking our shoes off and throwing
our clothes on the floor is very different from placing our shoes in front of the door and
folding our clothes away. And, while in that moment of folding our clothes away, paying
full attention to the folding of the clothes: the feel of the fabric, its weight and the colour.
When we bring respectful, loving attention to all that we are and all that we do, we –
and all things – feel most alive.

When we touch one thing with awareness, we touch all things. In his beautiful poem 'The Mistress of Vision', Francis Thompson writes 'All things by immortal power, Near or far, Hiddenly, To each other linked are. That thou canst not stir a flower Without Troubling of a Star'. These beautiful words encourage us to tread gently with ourselves, each other and our earth. What we do unto others, unto our earth and unto things, we do unto ourselves. Practising gratitude encourages greater care and kindness in our days. A sudden appreciation for our oneness with all life has the power to transform our experience of living from one moment to the next.

Living mindfully means living magically: being attuned to the subtle, delightful and inspiring nuances in our moment-to-moment lives. Indeed, our appreciation and full presence can transform any 'ordinary' moment into an extraordinarily delightful possibility.

Where there is love,
there is life.

Mahatma Gandhi

'I am Happy in This Moment'
EXERCISE

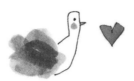

We can be very quick to say that we are unhappy, stressed or strained, yet there are so many moments, big and small, in our days in which we are deeply touched by joy. When we make it a habit to notice and mark these happy moments with our attention we not only feel the depth of our joy, we invite even more happiness into our lives through our own gratitude and mindful awareness.

I like to mark my happy moments with the simple words 'I am happy in this moment', smiling as I say these words either out loud or in my mind. This could be watching my puppy run through the garden chasing a stick, receiving a wonderful cuddle from a loved one, tucking into a warm and cosy bed, or drinking a nice cup of tea. You might feel happy listening to a particular piece of music, being in the presence of an old friend, or taking in a particular view.

I find that when I say the words 'I am happy in this moment' followed by a deep breath in and out, the moment is crystallised and honoured. I also find that I notice how many special, magical moments I do have, even on a day that might seem 'ordinary', for want of a better word!

So if you are seeking greater happiness in all your days, try marking and honouring all your happy moments with this these six little words:

'I am happy in this moment.'

I promise it will become a habit you'll keep and cherish for life.

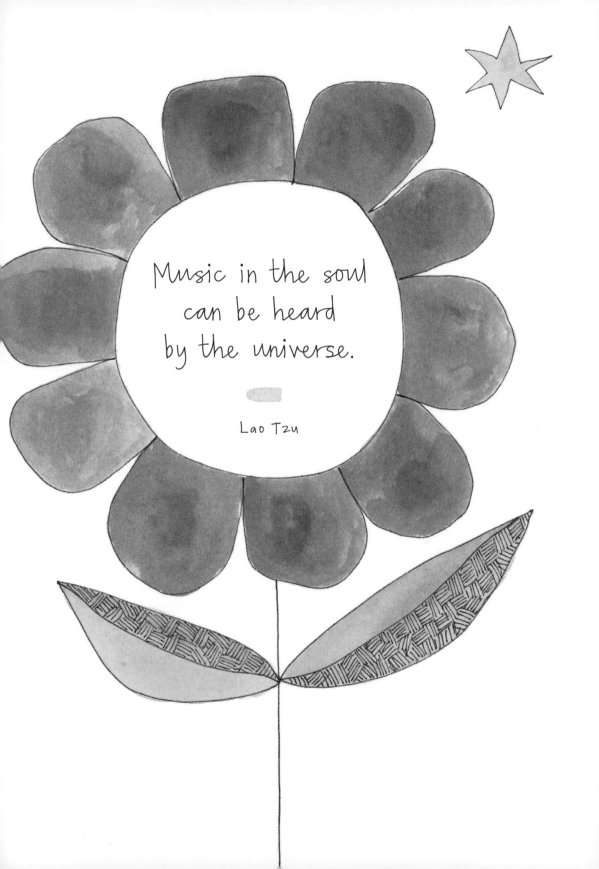

Music in the soul
can be heard
by the universe.

Lao Tzu

MAKING MAGIC —
EMBRACING JOY

'Magical living sounds wonderful,' you say, 'but I don't have any time to answer the calls of my spirit!' Where can we begin? I suggest to start small but to ask big questions. How might I soften my gaze upon life right now? What is working, well and good in my life at the moment? How could I better balance work, rest and play? When might it be appropriate for me to say no to others and yes to myself? Could I approach my responsibilities and demands with new eyes?

Identifying what feels dull, tired and lacklustre in our lives and creating room to sparkle is a gift we can give ourselves and those around us. We can mindfully assess how we feel about our chosen work, our relationships, our home environments, the way we eat and move our bodies, the various responsibilities that might be bestowed upon us, our hobbies, passions and recreational activities. While it is unrealistic to think that our days won't hold various challenges and surprises, and naturally vary in light and shade, with gratitude and grace we can gain instant inspiration when feeling ordinary or grumbly. I love reframing: 'I get to do this' rather than 'I have to do this'.

Time poverty has a lot to do with our mindset and emotional state. If we are stressed and strained, time compresses. Spaciousness and joy will elude us because living this way, we will never have enough time. If we are graceful and relaxed, we can nurture a more spacious, elastic relationship with time, sensing that time is always abundant and on our side. When it comes to nurturing our spirits, it is about making, not finding time in daily life. As we have explored, prioritising the care of our inner sparkles is not selfish or indulgent; it is essential for our health and wellness. When we nurture our spirits we may live meaningful, energised lives, lives that deeply nourish and fulfil us.

Be creative with your wants, needs and desires in the context of your daily life, and be courageous when you see room for positive changes to be made. In my book *The Art of Gratitude* there is an exercise in which we draw a line down the centre of a piece of paper, listing our daily 'pleasures' on one side, our 'chores' on the other. This telling exercise requires our honesty, time and attention. What parts of our daily lives do we perceive and experience as pleasures, which parts do we see as chores? Once we complete our lists we are instantly able to get a bigger, clearer picture of our lives as we are currently living them. We can identify with the daily things that grow our joy, and those that dull our sparkle. We can then mindfully reassess whether it is our mindsets that need refreshment, our agendas that need reworking, or, in most cases, both! It is a joy to work with this list, increasing our 'P's for pleasure and minimising our 'C's for chores, drawing on our instinct and emotional intelligence to problem solve, innovate and redesign our lives in congruence with our innermost needs and ideals. Rather than expending our precious energy fighting what is tired and old, we are called to get busy welcoming in what is right and new!

When we ask ourselves big questions regularly, tuning in to what actually matters to us and brings us joy, we begin to make daily, short-term decisions in alignment with our spirits and our bigger picture, long-term goals. We needn't ever be overwhelmed, thinking that we have to make lots of enormous changes all of a sudden. Simply by choosing to prioritise the nurturing of our sparkles in daily life, day by day, year by year, we find ourselves living lives in harmony with our values and dreams. We begin to feel all the more empowered, fulfilled, courageous and content.

Magical living encompasses all the things we do. When we choose to touch all parts of our lives with attention, appreciation and love, our lives give back to us with abundant joy and inspiration. Make constant daily effort to rise up and match the frequency of the joyous energy you want to feel. Let's be what we are looking for.

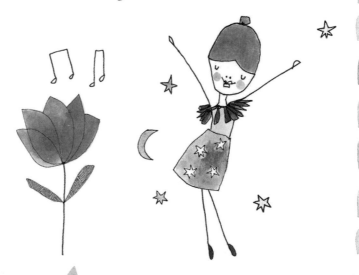

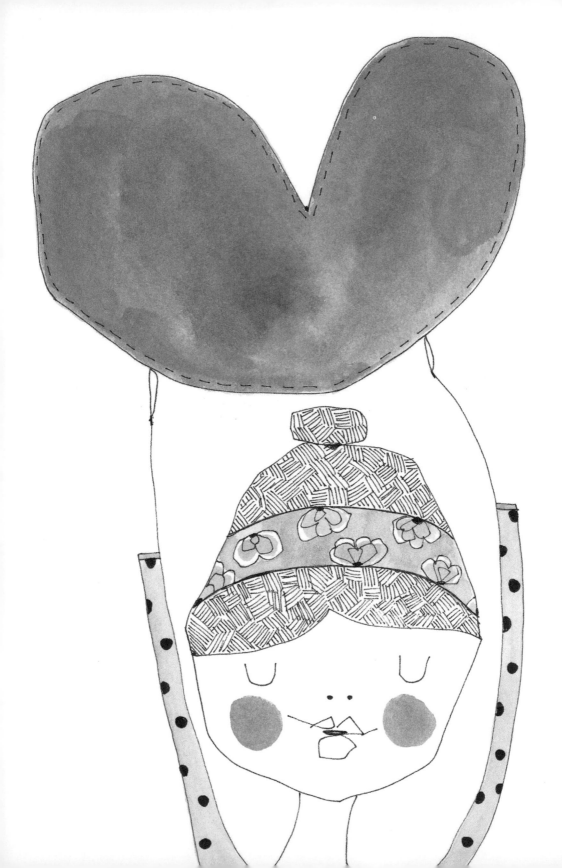

SUCCESS IS NOT THE
KEY TO HAPPINESS.
HAPPINESS IS THE
KEY TO SUCCESS.
IF YOU LOVE WHAT
YOU ARE DOING, YOU
WILL BE SUCCESSFUL.

Albert Schweitzer

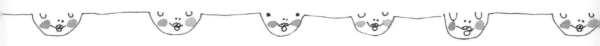

WHEN FEELING LACKLUSTRE

A very important part of sparkle-care is paying attention to the wise, encouraging messages we constantly receive. Profound invitations for healing and flourishing can open up to us through the challenging seasons and states of being in our lives, bringing us the perspective and motivation we seek. With self-awareness we begin to realise that our spirits will tickle us in all manner of ways to get our attention if we ignore them, and illuminate our forward paths faithfully if we allow them.

We are not alone when we long for more meaning, more connection and more kindness in our lives. This longing for more is collective. The challenging states that we experience personally are known and felt by all human beings in all manner of ways. When our spirits seek deeper and more sustaining experiences our yearning can present itself in different, often challenging states of being. Restlessness, depression, conflict, disharmony; even pain and physical illness can be understood and tended to as very important messages from deep within. While lacklustre states and experiences can be unpleasant to endure, they are valuable calls to tend to our spiritual wellbeing – to explore, nourish and nurture ourselves as deeply and lovingly as possible. When viewed not as failings but rather as invitations to look more deeply, love more deeply, or choose differently, we may experience and explore lacklustre states as gateways to our bliss.

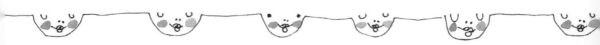

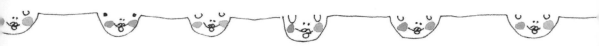

Our negativity, cynicism and sarcasm can be our world-weariness at play. A disconnection from the mystery of life. A call for us to return to gratitude, humility and grace. Our irritability and grumpiness can be an expression of unfulfilled desires of our souls; invitations to balance rest and play in our daily lives; to dial down our seriousness and reconnect with joy and nurture our sense of humour. Our fatigue might be directing us to reassess the ways we use and expend our precious personal energy. Perhaps we need to better protect our personal boundaries to nurture our vitality? Perhaps we are not enjoying the work that we do, and are being encouraged to make positive change? It might be a call to observe and workshop relationships and circumstances that deplete us. In any case, tiredness is a wonderful call for us to slow down, tread lightly and go gently with our spirits.

Our self-pity might be best understood as disconnection from our own power. A call to take responsibility for the thoughts we think and the choices we make, and an invitation to reconnect with our deep inner strength and courage. We are often quick to feel victimised by our circumstances, failing to acknowledge just how much we can do about them! Empowering ourselves through conscious and selective thinking, exploring our self-healing, self-soothing powers and activating our creativity are great ways to face and combat our self-pity. Similarly, our self-doubt can be read as a disconnection from our intuition. Doubting ourselves invites us to reconnect with our immense inner wisdom, and to surrender to faith in being divinely guided and protected through life. With such magical awareness we awaken to infinitely greater love and support, and our self-belief and confidence naturally blossom.

Physical and emotional clutter that crowds us can be taken as a call to see what we cannot let go of in our lives. How might we be seeking to fill real internal voids or needs by jam-packing our calendars or accruing more things? Noticing our cluttered thoughts, agendas or spaces invites us to consciously create breathing room in our lives and enjoy greater peace and flow. By honestly reassessing our values and priorities, we are able to embark on healing and refreshing decluttering journeys that can radically elevate our spirits and profoundly improve our daily lives.

Rather than feel ruffled by feelings of dissatisfaction, we can courageously accept the call that our dissatisfaction presents to us and design our lives in better alignment with our innermost values and desires. When we are dissatisfied we intuitively know that there is more to life waiting for us. Our spirits are encouraging us to move towards the bliss and joy we sense is possible for us. When we live our own lives in our own way with a firm focus on what truly matters to us, not what matters to those whom we might wish to please or impress, we find the deep and lasting satisfaction we seek. Stepping up to dissatisfaction with action is a truly satisfying course.

Another common and confounding feeling we can face is a sense of purposelessness in life. We may question why we are here, and what the point of our lives really might be. In my eyes, experiencing a sense of purposelessness is our invitation to acknowledge that we are significant; that our spirits matter; and that our contribution matters. It is a call for us to connect and reconnect with the miracle of life and our oneness with life and each other. Rumi reminds us that in being human we are not just a drop in the ocean, we are the entire ocean in a drop. The entire universe is within us, empowering and fortifying us with magical energy, moment to moment. Find out what it is that ignites your inner sparkle by noticing when you feel joy. Allow your joy to illuminate the purpose of your life's energy. By doing what we love and doing it lovingly while caring for others and our earth, we swiftly reconnect with a sense of meaning and purpose in our lives.

In addition to calling upon and cultivating our emotional intelligence to fortify and enliven our sparkles, balance our moods and refresh our states of mind, it is important to nurture ourselves physically in order to support the wellness of our spirits. Our bodies are after all our mind and spirit homes on earth, and when our bodies are nourished our sparkles may flourish all the more. Choose quality, natural whole foods, drink ample fresh water, enjoy fresh air, digital detoxes, time in nature, healthy, uplifting personal rituals, and rest and relaxation. Daily self-care practices such as these can swiftly, deeply restore our freshness and clarity for life. Should uneasy states of being become stubborn or persistent, you may wish to explore the possibility of biochemical imbalances, food intolerances, allergies or compromised gut health. These physical things can directly and profoundly affect the mental, spiritual and emotional states we experience.

While some food cravings are due to biochemical imbalances in the body worth exploring in terms of dietary change and supplementation, powerful metaphysical explanations may also shed light on food cravings. Sweet cravings often manifest when we lack sweetness in our lives. We might ask ourselves, 'How can we experience more sweetness and joy in our lives?' Junk-food cravings can call us to heal our self-sabotaging habits. We might ask ourselves, 'How can we feel more worthy of our own love and care?' Overeating can be our way of protecting ourselves from pain by 'stuffing down' our challenging thoughts and feelings. We might ask ourselves, 'How can we support ourselves to courageously see and rewrite our stories?' Under-eating can call us to appreciate and care for ourselves with true tenderness and compassion. We might gently ask, 'How can we see our own strength and beauty? How can we fall more in love with ourselves?' When we quieten down our busy thoughts, tune in and ask our bodies what they truly want and need, we may receive profound intuitive guidance. Concerns around food are often calls to explore the hungry parts of our emotional bodies that need our honesty, compassion and attention. We can accept such invitations courageously, learning to satisfy our real hunger for life in nurturing ways that allow our spirits to blossom.

Our spirits are always at the helm. When we nurture them lovingly, all things in and around us seem to fall into place. When our spirits are nurtured, issues we face that once seemed extremely complex can all of a sudden become clearer to understand and simpler to resolve. Hurries or worries that once seemed insurmountable can be illuminated and present themselves for transformation. We are in this life together, learning, growing and changing. We can support ourselves and each other to practise true self-care and self-love and, in doing so, find our sparkles.

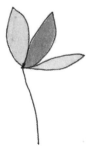

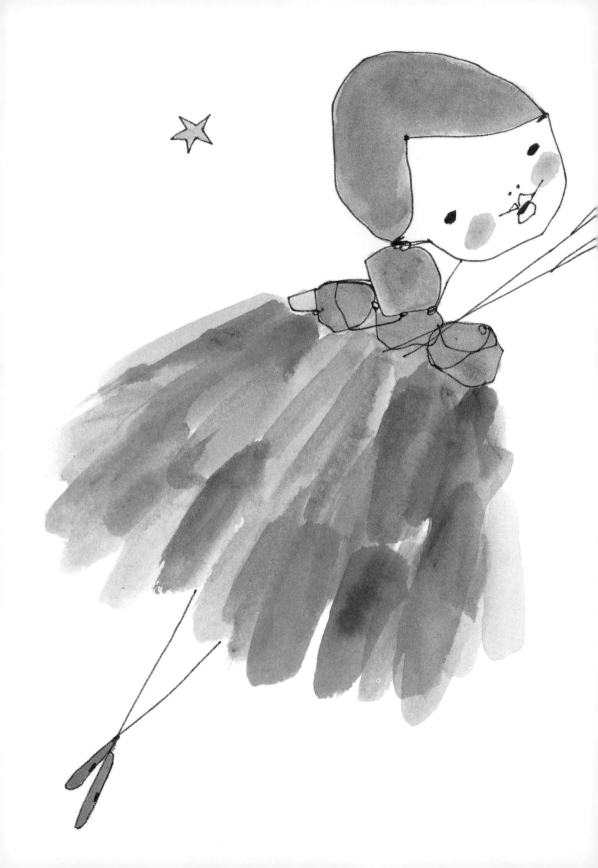

WHY DO YOU
STAY IN PRISON,
WHEN THE DOOR IS
SO WIDE OPEN?

Rumi

Why not feel

RADIANT

BLISSFUL

OPENHEARTED

CONNECTED

INSPIRED

ENCHANTED

FULFILLED?

m

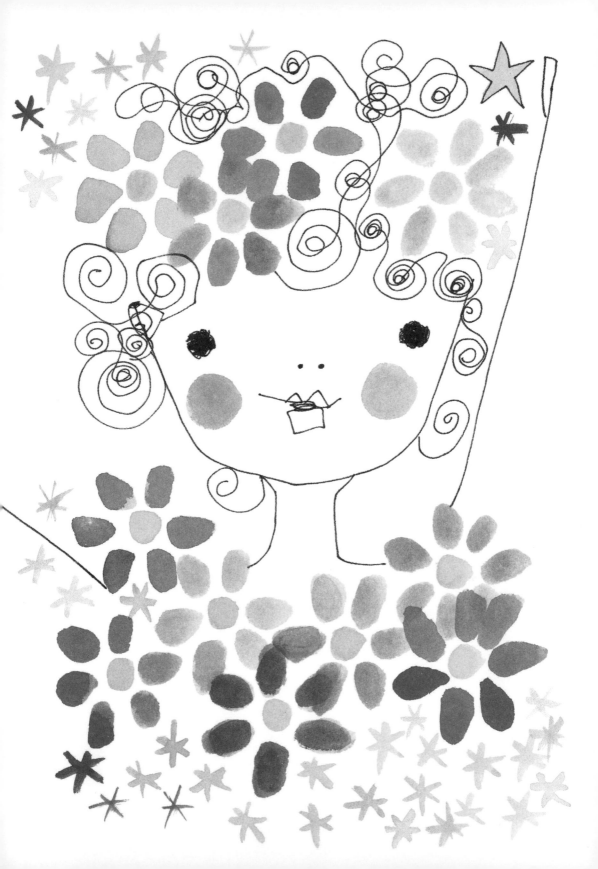

Stress and Sparkling

Some kinds of stress are natural, necessary, motivating and even positive, such as the mounting adrenaline we feel before we take a test or run a race. Positive stress helps us leap into action and perform at our best. Yet acute or what can become constant underlying negative stress can debilitate us, diminishing our glow and affecting us in ways we might not even appreciate. Learning to meet, greet and manage our stress is truly empowering. Rather than seeing stress as something we should eliminate altogether (as this is not humanly possible), we can learn to identify and understand our stress. We can draw on simple, savvy ways to manage it before it manages us!

Stress causes inflammation at a cellular level, compromising our immune systems, contributing to disease and reducing our overall mental and physical vitality. When stressed we breathe shallowly, radically decreasing the amount of cleansing, nourishing oxygen that can reach our cells. When stressed we are susceptible to experiencing indigestion and stomach upsets, even challenges with our menstrual cycles, skin, sleep cycles, moods and more. Emotionally, our stress can cause us to lose precious perspective, patience and peace.

Stress is the launch of various bodily processes instigated by our brain's perception that we are under attack. According to Mithu Storoni, neuroscientist and author of the book *Stress Proof*, 'psychosocial' stress is our biggest stressor today: that is, feeling threatened by other people. In the past our greatest stressors were the wild animals that could eat us alive, or the savage environmental conditions that could jeopardise our livelihood. These days, however, it is our fellow human beings causing us the most angst. Think of the comparison or competition we can feel with one another, the sense of judgement we can feel exposed to day to day, or the bullying and power plays that generally colour unsupportive, unhealthy relationships. Simply by choosing kindness and compassion for ourselves and each other we can actively minimise a great deal of this psychosocial stress, person by person, day by day. Yet until everyone chooses to ride this wave of kindness together, we are very wise to have some stress-savvy tricks up our sleeves for interpersonal stresses and stressful challenges of all kinds.

Identifying and naming our stress empowers us. The hardest part is when we are thinking or acting out of stress and don't acknowledge it, or when we are not attuned to what is actually stressing us out and forge ahead without any self-awareness. Simply taking a look at our lives in the present moment and saying or writing down for ourselves 'I am stressed now because . . .' is part of bringing our stress into the light. Once our stressors are flood-lit and named, they can become far less scary, abstract or amorphous. At this powerful point we can work with our stress, tending to ourselves with self-soothing, self-sustaining acts of self-care.

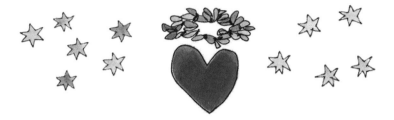

When we feel our stress levels rising we are immediately called to choose a personalised remedy with love. Do we need some fresh air or a few long, deep breaths? Do we need a tall glass of fresh water or a soothing cup of herbal tea? Do we need to talk to a good friend or confidant? Do we need to stop ruminating and pour our focus into a crossword, some dance steps or a creative project? Do we need to have an early night, enjoy some yoga or have a massage? Do we need to have a laugh or practise a little mindfulness? With so many options at hand to soothe and comfort ourselves moment to moment, we needn't feel helpless in the face of stress. We can choose from a joyous list of relaxing options that soothe, balance and refresh us. We are all works in progress, learning every day. Learning to see stress for what it is helps empower us to take it out of the darkness and into the light for healing and transformation.

It is wonderful to note that the better we become at following our bliss, delighting our senses and embracing our sparkles, the more resilient to stress we naturally become. When we love and approve of ourselves, others' opinions of us become just that: opinions, not definitions. When we each nourish and nurture our own sparkles, others' shines cannot take away from our own, nor can our shine threaten others. When we take the time to know our spirits, we can make decisions in support of our ongoing health and happiness. By nurturing our sparkles we're already going a great way towards managing, reducing and transforming any challenges we may meet in this life.

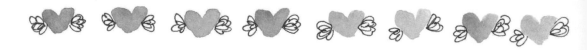

SPARKLE NURTURE FOR HIGHLY SENSITIVE SOULS

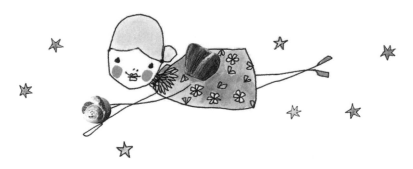

We are all sensitive beings but some of us are more sensitive than others. Sometimes we don't even realise what this means, or how to care for ourselves. Instead we berate ourselves for being weak, overly emotional, too soft, possibly even consider ourselves unequipped for relationships and experiences of all kinds! Feeling this way we might retreat and wrap ourselves in cotton wool, concerned about surviving life's knocks both great and small. Yet this is no way to live life to the fullest. We can be highly sensitive people but nurture our sparkles in a way that we feel protected, strengthened and guided by our sensitivity, rather than hindered or weakened by it.

Highly sensitive people move through life picking up on the energy of people, places and things with a particular immediacy and intensity. Intuitive, compassionate and empathic, they can often sense how others are thinking and feeling. They feel the energy of places, sometimes even picking up on stories past, present and future. When those around them are sad or unwell, highly sensitive people feel along with, or even take on the states of, others: a lived reality that can become very tiring and confusing for a highly sensitive person. It can become very difficult for highly sensitive people to feel their personal boundaries – to discern where their own thoughts and feelings end and others' begin.

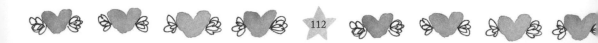

Bright lights, loud, overwhelming people and sounds, crowds and confrontation are just some things that can ruffle a highly sensitive soul, causing feelings of stress and overwhelm. While some of us enjoy noise and chaos, life can simply feel too loud, too bright and too nerve-racking at times for those of us who are highly sensitive. Sometimes we don't even know why we feel so emotional, tired or overcome in certain situations, but we do. We feel life deeply on all levels.

Highly sensitive souls are called to practise extra self-care in daily life and honour their spirit's calls to feel safe and grounded. Extra rest and downtime is very important for highly sensitive people, who are mostly introverted by nature. Unlike extroverts who recharge their batteries through socialising and adventurous action, introverts replenish their energy by going within and taking quiet time out to rest their minds, bodies and spirits. Soothing mindfulness meditations, self-strengthening positive affirmations and protective visualisations are particularly supportive for highly sensitive people, bringing balance to both their mindset and nervous system.

Mindful awareness of triggering situations such as crowded environments, overbearing personalities, horrifying movies or devastating news footage can help the highly sensitive person to take appropriate and necessary measures to comfort and support themselves in daily life. Limiting or avoiding exposure to such influences while maintaining a sense of connection to others and to life is essential. Exploring the protective, strengthening powers of crystals such as citrine, hematite and black tourmaline can be most helpful, along with essential oils including grounding frankincense on the soles of the feet, or lavender oil applied to the wrists in times of stress. Flower essences and homeopathic remedies may also provide extra comfort and support for the highly sensitive soul when needed, and are a joy to discover.

We can never assume to understand exactly how somebody else sees or feels in the world. Being honest with ourselves and others about our feelings can help us to design lives that support our unique personalities and spirits. Be respectful of yourself as a highly sensitive person, or of highly sensitive people with whom you share your world. Highly sensitive people can sparkle very brightly and, with the right nurturing, may experience and share their immense wisdom, light and love.

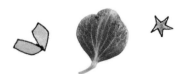

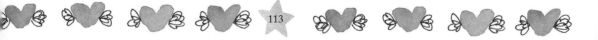

NORMALITY IS
A PAVED ROAD:
IT'S COMFORTABLE
TO WALK, BUT
NO FLOWERS
GROW ON IT.

Vincent van Gogh

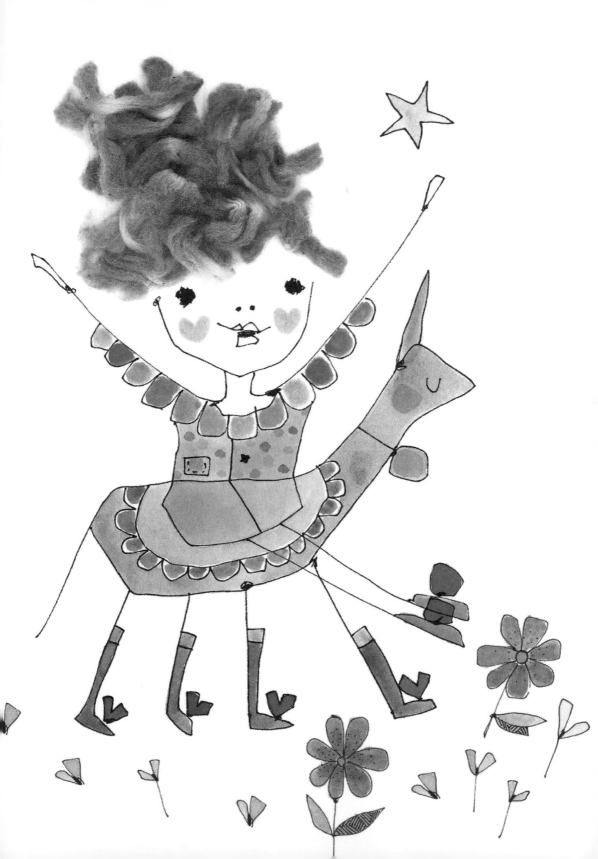

CLOUD THOUGHTS MEDITATION

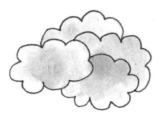

Slowing my busy thoughts now
I deepen my breathing.
Breathing in and breathing out
completely, deeply, slowly.

On my next in-breath
I let a thought come to mind,
whatever it may be.
I let myself think this thought fully.
Inhaling right to the top of my breath now
I pause and let my thought go, seeing it float up
and out through the top of my head like a cloud.
I see my thought floating,
weightlessly, effortlessly,
up, out and away.

On my next in-breath I let another thought come to mind,
whatever it may be.
Perhaps it is a stressful thought.
Perhaps it is a happy thought.
Perhaps it is a funny thought.
Perhaps it is a tender thought.

Inhaling right to the top of my breath now
I pause and let this thought go too, seeing it float up
and out through the top of my head like a cloud —
floating, weightlessly, effortlessly,
up and away.

Now there are two clouds of my thoughts,
floating free in space.
Might there be any other thoughts I wish to send
up and away while I am here?
I take a moment to think about any other thoughts I have now,
letting them go, one by one
and seeing them float up, out and away.

Flowing with each inhale and exhale now,
I notice that each and every thought is like a cloud.
Floating in and floating out.
Changing and shifting.

Nothing is forever.
The sky is never the same.
I am free to think my thoughts.
To choose and change my thoughts.
To let them grow and let them go.
Seeing my thoughts like clouds in the sky
I breathe on, open, light and free.

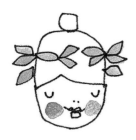

Seeing my thoughts
like passing clouds in the sky
I breathe on,
open, light and free.

M

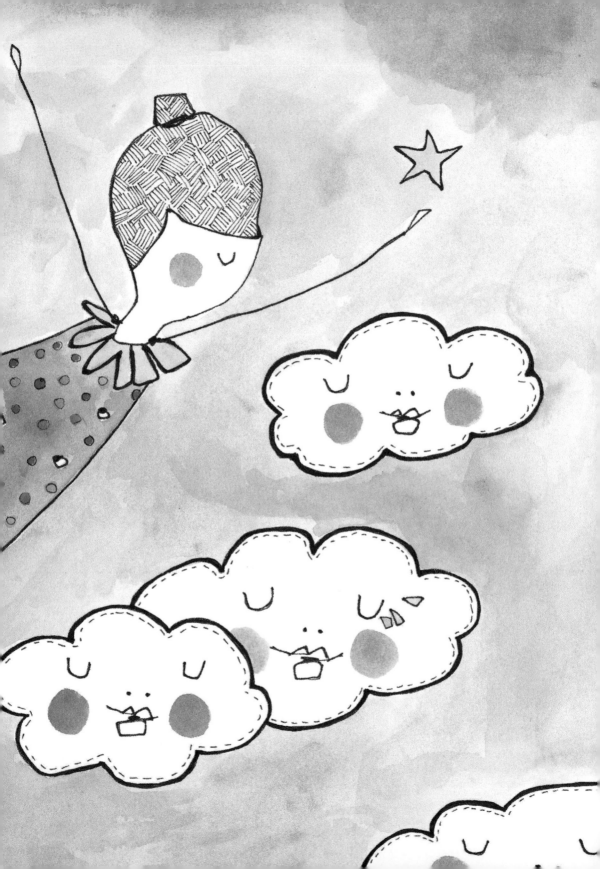

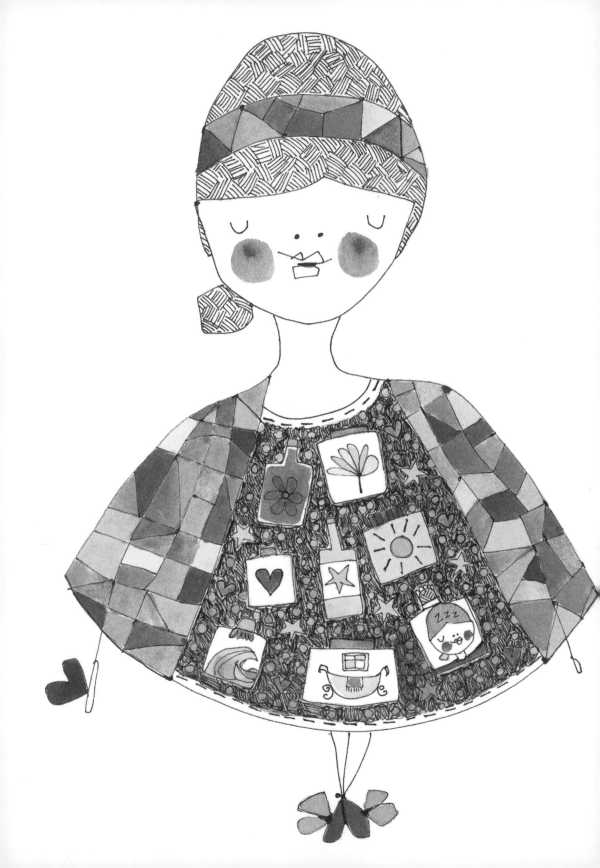

SELF-HEALING MAGIC

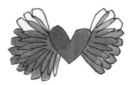

Too often we give our power away. We expect other people or other things
to heal us, complete us or fill us up. Yet when we see at last that we are
home in our tremendous power, that we always have been and always will
be, we can learn to trust in ourselves and the perfect order of nature.
We can touch a kind of inner power, peace and joy that we deserve to know
yet are rarely, if ever, 'taught' to access. Indeed, we all have the capacity
to soothe, comfort and inspire ourselves and, in doing so, experience truly
sustainable, healing and fortifying energy as long as we live. It is important
to note that I refer here to more general and milder feelings of depression,
anxiety and malaise. Those suffering more acutely may find that self-
healing practices can work in wonderful harmony with the recommendations
of their trusted health professionals.

Sharpening our emotional mind–body intelligence and realising the immensity of our
own healing power could have profound and life-changing consequences. If each one of
us were to awaken to our own magical, self-healing potential and come to know simple,
true comfort and happiness from within, we would be able to step aside from the constant
seeking of bliss and into the lived experience of it. What if we weren't anxious and
depressed but rather world-weary as a natural response to modern life? What if to regain
our sparkles we were to simply heed the calls of our spirits, courageously taking small steps
to begin to live more magical lives? What if we were to have faith in our own capacity to
restore, soothe and balance ourselves? Would we still feel the need to consult others about
what might be 'wrong' with us and seek to be fixed?

The truth is that we naturally possess healing wisdom and power within us – pure instinct;
deep intuition. In the wise and poignant words of Alsatian theologian Albert Schweitzer,
'The doctor of the future will be oneself . . . Every patient carries his or her own doctor
inside . . .' If we quieten down and listen in, we always know the answers. In the instances

in which external support or intervention are genuinely warranted, we will most certainly know to seek help. Otherwise, it is the loving, tender and unconditionally respectful relationship we nurture with ourselves that heals and fortifies us for life, and which is free and available to us, moment to moment.

When we consider nurturing our tremendous self-healing and self-sustaining powers, it is helpful to see our inner sparkle as our life force. All thoughts and acts born from fear deplete our life force, dull our sparkle, estrange us from one another and thieve our energy. When we are judgemental, hurried, fearful and worried we deplete our life force. When we eat mindlessly or dishonour our minds and bodies with carelessness and unkindness, our lights dwindle. In contrast, thoughts and acts born from love strengthen our life force, nourish our sparkle, bring us healing and expand our energy. Rest, self-care and self-compassion grow our inner strength and self-worth, leading to positive thoughts and choices, and gentler and easier living. The more confident and peaceful we feel, the more we sparkle. Rumi suggested that if we want to feel more alive, love is our truest health.

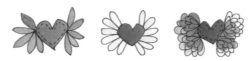

We all possess little and big darknesses within that call for our compassion and care. Indeed, the art of self-healing calls us to bring our loving attention to the parts of ourselves and our lives that need our special honesty, attention and light: parts that might be dark, lonely, detached or foggy. This can be both uneasy and confronting for us to do. Sometimes we worry so much about what we will find when we look more deeply into our inner worlds, but, unlike the proverbial monster under the bed waiting to terrify us, we can expect to be met with the tenderness, realness and integrity of who we truly are. Our perfectly imperfect, vulnerable, lovable and whole selves. By calling on courage and remembering that we are not alone in feeling our feelings; that we share this life with all other feeling human beings; that life is naturally composed of light and shade, ups and downs, we may cultivate the patience and self-compassion we so deeply crave and deserve.

You might like to visualise yourself as having an inner apothecary in which the right medicine for your mind, body and spirit is always at hand. This medicine might be rest. It might be laugher. It might be time out. It might be movement or connection with others. It might be helping somebody else on their path, having a quiet bath, taking some herbs or enjoying a nourishing meal, taking a walk in nature or savouring a moment of mindful presence. Allow yourself to gently explore healing possibilities and tend to yourself with love, tenderness and care. The empowerment you will experience by allowing yourself to know your own answers is a gift. You will find yourself to be more self-sufficient, intuitive, robust and magical than you could ever have imagined.

4-7-8 Breathing Technique

This is a wonderful breathing technique that I learned while listening to Dr Andrew Weil deliver an address on health and wellbeing. It is a wonderful resource when feeling restless at night or when anxious, stressed or strained. We can practise this simple technique by getting ourselves into a comfortable standing position, arms hanging gently by our sides, and exhaling fully.

We breathe in for four counts, then hold our breath for seven counts and then, with the fullest exhale possible, expel all the air from our lungs to the count of eight.

Beginning again, we inhale to the count of four then hold our breath for seven counts, and with the biggest, huffiest and puffiest exhale possible, expel all our breath out until our lungs feel utterly empty again, to the count of eight. We repeat this exact sequence for another two rounds to make a total of four rounds, and we are done.

We may feel a little tingly, perhaps even a little light-headed during our first practices of this exercise. This is a sign that our cells are being fully oxygenated at last. Often we breathe in very shallow ways, and our bodies can be a little surprised by a flood of wonderful, fresh air circulating within! I recommend practising this breathing exercise twice daily, ideally morning and night, as instructed by Dr Weil.

For your first month begin only with one sequence of this four-round exercise at a time. After a month of practice, and only if you feel comfortable, you can increase to a maximum of two sequences (that is, eight rounds in total).

What I find practising this simple, swift technique is that I am gifted with a lasting sense of relaxation and peace: a little like a yoga session rolled into a short, simple sequence of breaths. It is a wonderful technique to draw upon for daily resilience and stress relief, to assist with managing cravings, to energise ourselves in the morning and help us fall asleep at night.

Over time Dr Weil suggests that this technique can provide real marked health benefits, including lowering increased heart rates and high blood pressure, improving digestion and even treating anxiety. Simply remember to inhale, hold and exhale to the counts of 4-7-8, and enjoy the wonderful, healing benefits this magical technique can offer.

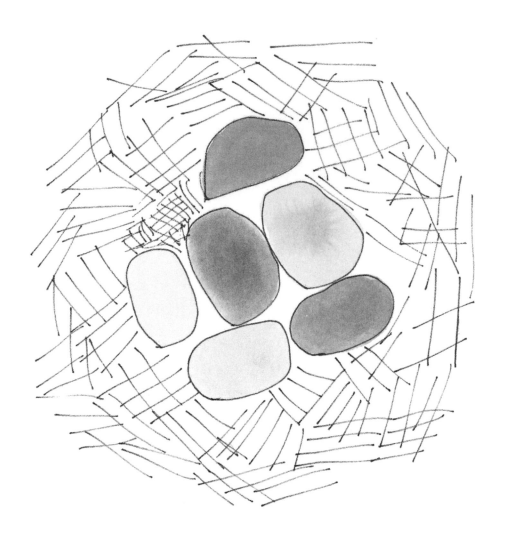

There are only two ways to live your life.
One is as though nothing is a miracle.
The other is as though everything is a miracle.

Albert Einstein

PRESENT-MOMENT MAGIC IN A DIGITAL AGE

The incredible rise of technology, especially social media, has meant
that many of us are existing in two realms in any given moment.
We are experiencing the present moment in physical time and space,
while busy working out how to best represent it to others through words
and pictures in the virtual world. Never before have we documented
and shared our lives so obsessively and instantaneously.

Representing our lives through social media can be an exciting and creative experience,
but it can also create immense distraction and anxiety. We are busy putting our lives on
show, and not only to those with whom we share our physical world but to innumerable
strangers in all places.

Many of us now find it hard to have a beautiful experience and keep it to ourselves.
The food we eat, the views we see, the trips we take, the intimate moments of connection
we are a part of. Of course, there is real joy in sharing our lives with others, but we are
called to intuit a happy medium in which we are present in the here and now, and are able
to hold our magic in deeply personal ways, just for ourselves. We are called to be still and
present with ourselves and others with whom we share our real world. To breathe life in
and hold it attentively, respectfully and completely.

Kahlil Gibran was famous for writing that we should 'Travel and tell no one. Live a true
love story and tell no one. Live happily and tell no one. People ruin beautiful things'.
While his final four words here could be read as a comedic addition, they could also be
a painfully accurate portrait of the often conflicted relationship that we can have with
our own human condition.

Sadly, as we count the comments and likes rolling in from the ether, we are taken away
from our here and now. We expose ourselves to all manner of energy from the outer
world – good, bad and in between. Even though we seem to seek it, none of us needs

to feel beholden to others' good opinions or approval of us. If we are living loving, authentic lives, we needn't exhaust our energy reserves wondering how liked or likeable we are. Our lives needn't become showreels, and needn't necessarily be publicised to such an extent. The role of social media in our modern lives is no small or frivolous matter. Our addiction to our devices is creating distance in our relationships with ourselves, each other and the natural world around us.

Next time you have a precious experience, close your eyes and channel your energy inward. Dive into the sensations you are feeling in your body, the magic that you feel circulating within and around you. Notice small details and be present. You'll find a whole new level of magic and fulsome delight available to you when you shift your focus away from all other distractions – away from the need to report back and have others bear witness – and immerse yourself right back into the immediacy and intimacy of your very own life and senses. Herein lies a simple, wonderful way to nurture your inner sparkle in daily life.

Another important aspect of technology, connectivity and wellness has to do with the very precious times just after we wake in the morning and right before we fall asleep at night. Do not miss these sacred moments in your day, moments in which your spirit is suspended in the magical space between dreaming and waking. Try switching off from technology an hour or so before you go to sleep, and refrain from activating your devices as soon as you wake up in the morning. Instead, use these magical moments to reflect, journal, listen to beautiful music, meditate or potter, mindful activities that invite your full presence and awaken your spirit.

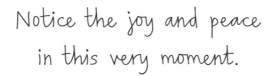

Notice the joy and peace
in this very moment.

M

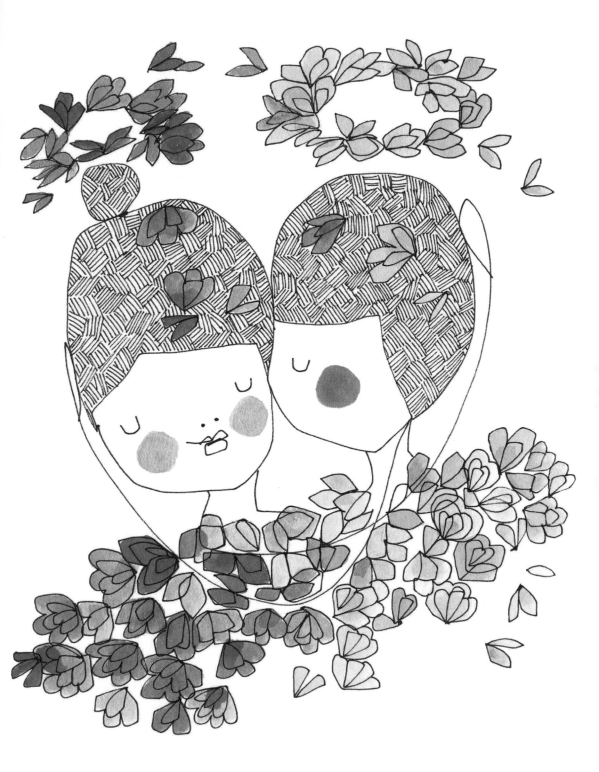

THE JOY OF EFFORT

There is true magic and sparkling joy to be found in the effort we make
and the work that we do. Often we begrudge effort as a kind of nuisance
or a means to an end, yet it is in our conscious, loving effort that true
fulfilment and reward can be found.

When we choose not to make effort in our lives we naturally feel tired, low and listless.
Our lack of care and disengagement with life and others clouds our joy. Effort, work
and participation are energising for our spirits and nourishing for our sparkles. When
we choose to be present and do things with love, all things, including so-called 'chores',
can become opportunities to feel happiness. Little moments we once passed by, too busy,
grumpy or impatient, can become moments of bliss.

Imagine yourself in a tiny remote cabin in the wilderness. You have only the most basic
essentials with which to live, none of the usual creature comforts. You've settled in for a
week, just to be. At night you light a candle after dark, sleeping with the moon and rising
with the sun. To light a warm fire you gather sticks from nature, pottering outside in the
elements rather than flicking on the air-conditioning. To gather produce you rely on what
grows around your cabin or what can be gifted or bought in the local community. There
is no home delivery available, no shops to visit close by. To pass time in your cabin you
explore, read, cook, sleep, stretch, daydream, reflect, perhaps even meditate. There's no
scrolling, no TV and no distraction.

In such an instance we see cause not only to celebrate simplicity and a life more attuned
to nature, we begin to notice the joy of effort. As we gather sticks outdoors we bend and
stretch and move our bodies. We breathe in the air and look up into the trees. We listen
to the sounds of the earth and feel the elements touch us. When we pick our fruit and
vegetables we connect with nature. We remind ourselves where our food truly comes
from, and have a chance to feel heightened gratitude for the abundance our earth bestows.
The act of eating becomes a magical privilege with which we prefer to take our time.
When we are gifted produce from others or source it locally we have a chance to support
community and feel part of something greater than ourselves. We build relationships to

fortify and uplift us. When we prepare our own food, simply and with full presence, we express our creativity and love, and participate actively in deeply nourishing ourselves.

Our habit of overcomplicating our lives with rumination, extreme busyness and clutter and then relying on convenience to minimise our work and effort can create an unnecessary unhappiness within us. Conversely, loving the work we do and making effort from our hearts in all parts of our lives ignites our sparkles. We find ourselves catapulted into the ecstasy of the present moment in which all things are just as they should be, and in which life is magical.

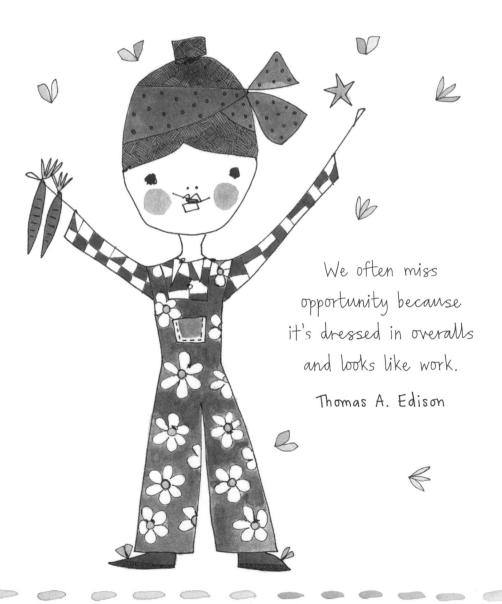

We often miss opportunity because it's dressed in overalls and looks like work.

Thomas A. Edison

Forming Constellations

People are not always as they seem. Things are not always as they seem. We are often very quick to make judgements about others based on superficial terms and with very little awareness. We can group people together, dismiss and judge others, even those of us who consider ourselves to be generally kind and generous people. When we label or judge people we simplify them, denying them their unique individuality, often even a chance. When we limit our friendships to those of a similar age or 'kind' as ourselves, we close our hearts to so many possibilities and so much magic along the way. We miss life-changing opportunities for connection, learning, love and friendship.

Meaningful bonds nourish us. When we connect meaningfully with each other we blossom, often in ways we could never even imagine or expect. Anais Nin wrote that each friend is a new world to discover, a new self. How magical this idea is to explore. Indeed, the more we open ourselves to joy and to learning, the more joyous and expansive we will feel. Some of us have been hurt and feel our hearts hardened to making new connections. Others are too busy and blind to others with whom we share our worlds. But then – a moment, a word, a touch, a tear, or some other event makes us feel our inner sparkles flickering within. Our hearts are reawakened to our true interconnectedness, and to the tenderness and perfect timing of grace.

When it comes to our wellbeing, loneliness is one of the most damaging states. Its effects have in recent studies been likened to those of smoking and obesity combined. Centenarians living in 'Blue Zones' around the world, those living happily and healthily into old age, are invariably living in community. ('Blue Zones' are areas around the world acknowledged for dietary and lifestyle practices that contribute to lower rates of illness and disease, greater overall health and longevity.)

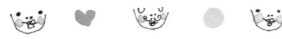

It is the very experience of belonging that they attribute to nourishing their joy, youthfulness and vitality. Knowing this, we are called to open our hearts and connect with each other. We often have no idea just how lonely others may be feeling, and we are called to practise generosity of spirit. We can reach out to others with our love and care, involve ourselves in community, include the excluded, and make time for each other. We can listen to each other's stories, sense our collective magic, and marvel in the inevitably common ground we share. As mindfulness teacher Sri Chinmoy asks, if our lives do not give joy to others, then how can we expect our hearts to give any joy to us? The more we disconnect, close our hearts and clip our wings, the less we live and the less we grow and sparkle. The more we listen, connect and grow together, the more reason we have to know our oneness and connect our sparkles into magnificent constellations. We shine all the more brightly when we shine together.

An old African proverb teaches that if we want to go fast, we should go alone. If we want to go far, we must go together. Our collective human suffering is our call to recalibrate and to go together. A call for community and togetherness. For kindness, compassion, imagination, faith and courage. Our longing is collective and, just as our problems are collective and shared, so our solutions will be. Supporting ourselves and each other to find magic in modern life and carve out space for listening, compassion and connection is key to the health and happiness of human beings and our planet – after all, we are all made of the same stardust. Together with our wise and ancient earth we are calling for faith, meaning and healing now; to experience the belonging and wellness we intuitively know is possible.

Our lives are ours to live, and they are best lived together. With open eyes, hearts and minds we can respect, welcome and elevate each other. We will find like-minded people on our path of joy; the people with whom we can truly celebrate the magic of life. If we find ourselves with more than we need, now we are being called to build bigger tables rather than taller fences. We are being encouraged to see ourselves and each other lovingly. A beautiful passage in the *Letter to the Hebrews* reads: 'Be not forgetful to entertain strangers, for thereby many have entertained angels unawares.' In my eyes, we are all angels incarnate on our journeys through life. We are all here unequivocally worthy, utterly loveable and timelessly divine.

SOMETIMES OUR
LIGHT GOES OUT,
BUT IS BLOWN AGAIN
INTO INSTANT FLAME
BY AN ENCOUNTER
WITH ANOTHER
HUMAN BEING.

Albert Schweitzer

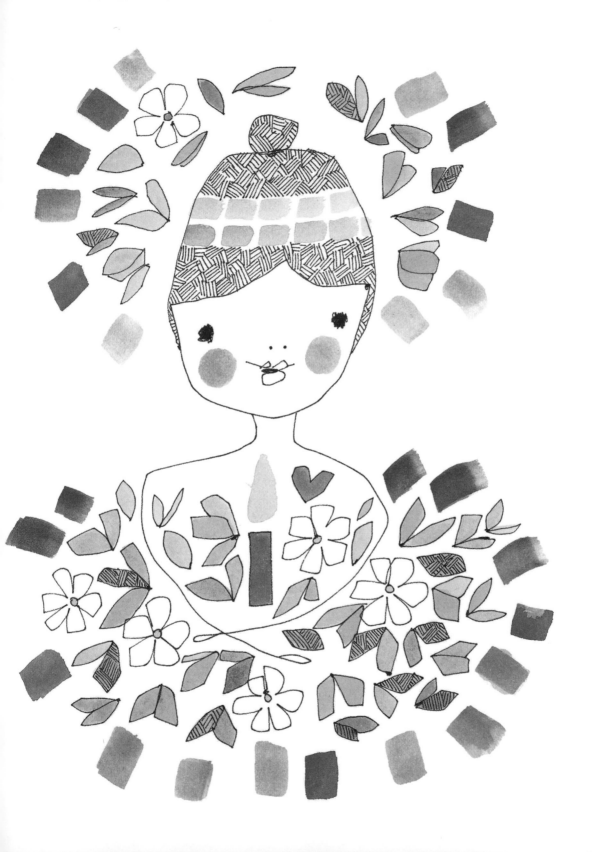

Wellness Prayer

We needn't consider ourselves to be religious in order to invite prayer into our lives.
In my eyes, prayers of love, gratitude and care are powerful, healing energetic
frequencies that do count, and do make a real difference to our own lives,
the lives of those with whom we share our world, and our beautiful earth.
Each day I love to enjoy this three-part prayer.

I begin by sitting comfortably and taking a few deep breaths.
I close my eyes and bring my hands into prayer pose,
positioning the base of my palms between my closed eyes.

First I send out a prayer for myself –
that I am happy and healthy.
That I am safe and loved.
I lift my hands up in the air gently and release them outward,
as if making an arc in the sky.

I take a deep breath in, and exhale out.
I return my hands to prayer pose again,
positioning the base of my palms between my closed eyes.

Next I send out a prayer for someone I know
who needs special love and support at this time.
I visualise this person safe and comforted.
I send them love and care.

I lift my hands up in the air and release them gently outward again,
making an arc in the sky.
I take another deep breath in, and exhale out.

Placing my hands together in the same way again
I now send out a prayer for our earth.
I see her brimming with life and health,
I see her radiant, magical and sparkling.

I send the earth love and healing, and I wish her peace and joy.
I breathe in and lift my hands up and out again,
making another arc in the sky to trace my exhale.

I am flowing with my breath now, breathing in and breathing out.

In this sacred space I take another few moments to relax.

Whenever I feel ready, I gently resume my day.

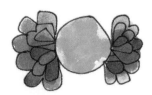

Climb the mountains and get their good tidings. Nature's peace will flow into you as sunshine flows into trees. The winds will blow their own freshness into you, and the storms their energy, while cares will drop away from you like the leaves of Autumn.

John Muir

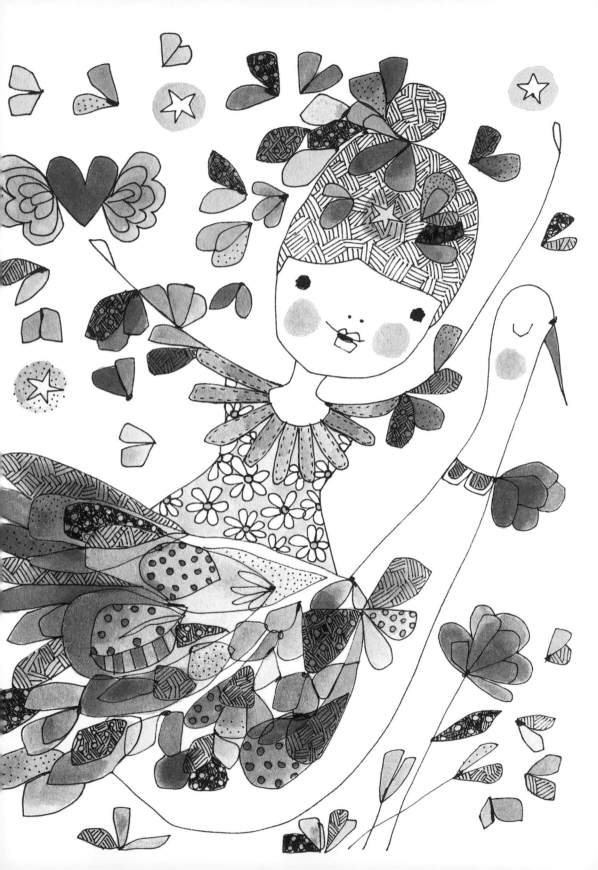

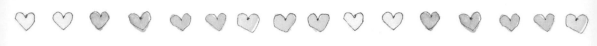

SPARKLING IN THE DARK

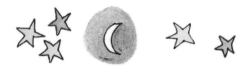

It takes a dark sky to enjoy the sparkle of a star. It takes pressure to cut the faces of a diamond so that it may sparkle. Our lives are inevitably coloured by changes in tone and mood. There are days we feel sparklier than others for reasons of all kinds, but even in our harder moments we give ourselves an enormous gift by remembering that we are still sparkling, always sparkling, simply by being alive.

In his beautiful book *No Mud No Lotus* Vietnamese Buddhist monk Thich Nhat Hanh teaches us that, like lotus flowers blossoming from the mud, we human beings may rise from the 'mud' of our lives, such as challenges, hardships or messy times we face, to flower magnificently. Indeed, a lotus blossom utilises and requires mud in order to thrive, flourish and grow all the more beautiful. While we are not born to suffer, life guarantees that we experience the lessons perfectly designed to enable us to grow. The most un-sparkly moments in our lives can take us to new heights of sparkling we never knew were possible.

Traditional Japanese ceramicists would fill cracks in their sculptures with gold. Rather than being viewed as mistakes, these gold-filled details were seen as essential parts of the object's originality and beauty — its unique magnificence. What if we were to visualise the cracks we have felt in our own lives, our own selves, filled with gold? To see them as precious parts of ourselves worthy of our loving appreciation? How differently we would see ourselves. The past is over, the future is not yet here. We are not damaged, we are healing. Life moves us forward with each moment.

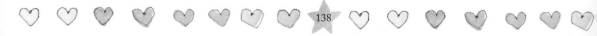

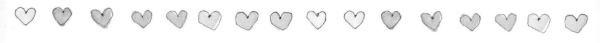

Each night the sparkling stars create a spectacular vision in the deep night sky. Each morning the sun rises to light up the dark. In this ever-steady rhythm we can take faith. When we possess a base awareness of being part of a greater movement of life in which we all effortlessly belong, in which the sunshine follows the rain, in which light eclipses the dark, in which we are together and at home in nature, we can find courage. Plato taught that courage is fear holding on a moment longer. Indeed, patience and reverence are qualities that see us through, allowing us like stars to sparkle in the darkness until the sun rises again.

When we appreciate the notion that all people and experiences come to us as divine lessons, we can train our minds to befriend personal challenges as opportunities for growth. Mindfulness meditation and mindful living practices help us to deal better with stress and frustration through cultivating inner balance and grace. From a calmer and more grounded position, we are able to access a sparkling solution for every 'problem', attuning ourselves to a higher intelligence that is always at play, guiding us to higher ground even if in seemingly circuitous ways.

When we open up to one another we inevitably realise that we share the same human feelings: hurts and doubts, hurries and worries. The same dark nights and desires of the soul. And while each one of us is unique, we share our essential humankind-ness. Our need to belong, our need to love and feel loved. When we practise kindness, respect and care for ourselves and each other at all times, including in the midst of our challenges, we find precious peace and inspiration. We connect meaningfully, not only with ourselves but with others who will love and support us, allowing us to feel the soothing care and understanding we seek during harder times.

When we sparkle, we glow with the richness of all that we have been, all that we are, and all that we can be. By welcoming all parts of ourselves and our stories back home with love each day, we may learn, grow and sparkle on.

Happiness is like a butterfly which, when pursued, is always beyond our grasp, but, if you will sit down quietly, may alight upon you.

Nathaniel Hawthorne

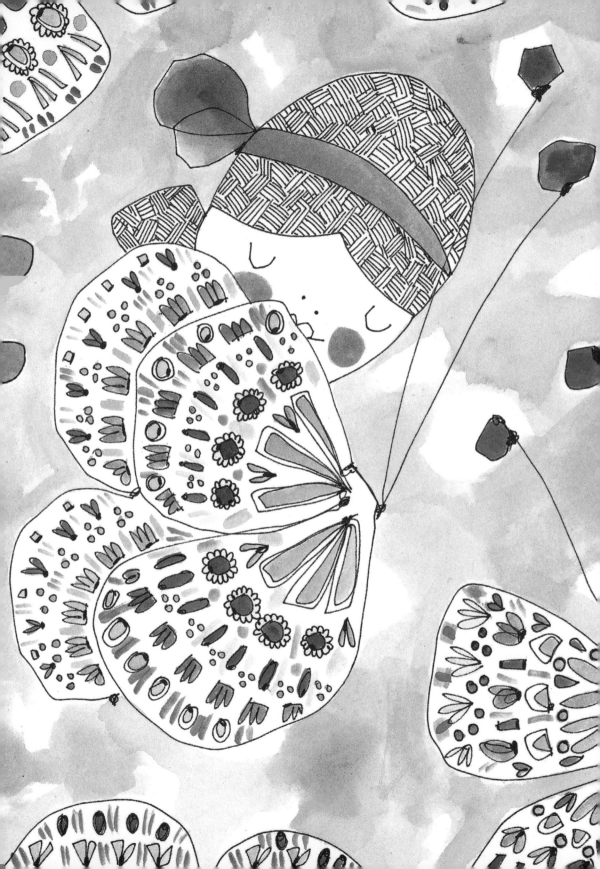

Finish each day and be done with it.
You have done what you could.
Some blunders and absurdities no
doubt crept in; forget them as soon
as you can. Tomorrow is a new day.
You shall begin it serenely and
with too high a spirit to be encumbered
with your old nonsense.

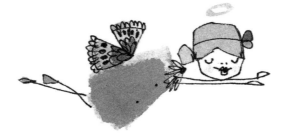

Ralph Waldo Emerson

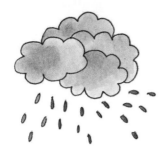
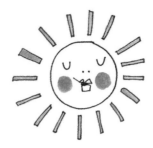

Rain to nourish our earth
Tears to soothe our spirits

Sunshine to light up our sky
Joy to fill our days

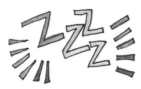
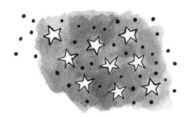

Storms that break and clatter
Challenges that wake us up to life

Stars that twinkle by night
Sparkling miracles, just like us

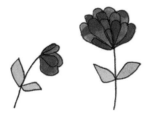

Flowers that grow with care
With love, we blossom

A butterfly from a chrysalis
Our potential for spectacular
transformation

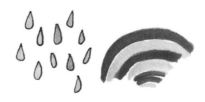

Leaves that change, fall and grow
Shedding old layers, we begin anew

Rainbows after rain
Keep courage - magic awaits

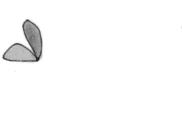

BE THE
RAINBOW
IN YOUR
OWN SKY!

m

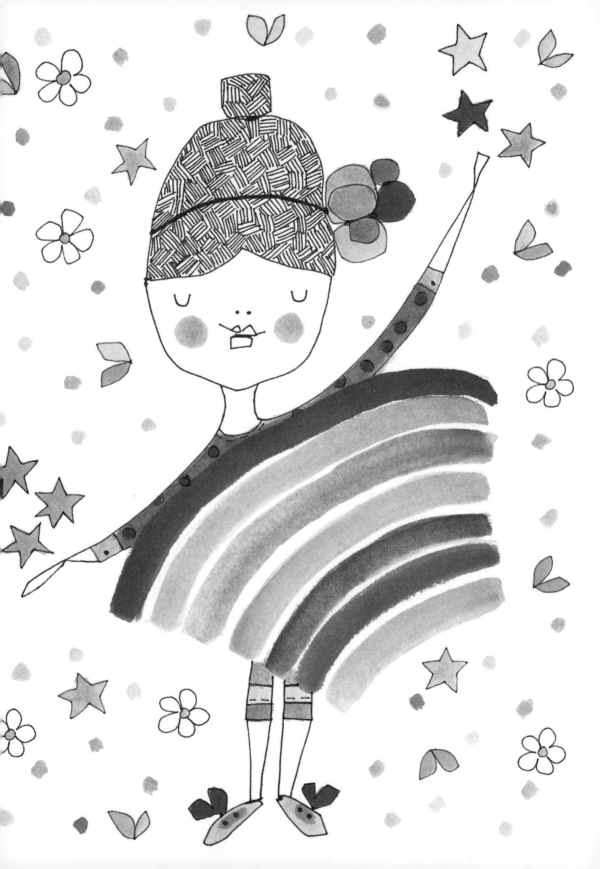

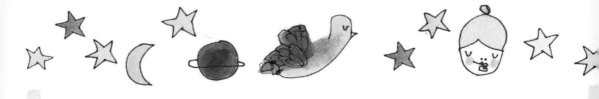

A Sparkle Revolution

The fast pace of this busy world can leave us breathless. Endless to-do lists and busy schedules tire and deplete us. We truly need rest but can't make time to be quiet! In the quiet moments we do have, we feel restless, distracted and overwhelmed. Despite promises made to us about shiny objects, bright and new, our 'things' do not make us happy in the lasting, fulfilling ways we wish they would. We can see that clutter, comparison and competition have been obstructing our joy. It's time for change now and we can feel it! In the words of Albert Einstein, 'The world will not evolve past its current state of crisis by using the same thinking that created the situation.' Indeed, we must think and see anew.

On a magical note, the current, collective awakening of which we are all a part is edging us closer to a revolution of spirit. We are awakening to the realisation that old 'civilised' systems we once accepted as normal and natural are no longer working for us or making us happy: systems concerning class and social status, beliefs around productivity and wealth accumulation, ideas about using our earth and her natural resources. More and more people are understanding the value of kindness, compassion and unity. More people are understanding that we need to care for our environment and are making daily effort to do so in simple but powerful ways, from riding a bike and recycling to avoiding plastics, composting and eating compassionately. More people are finding and choosing natural alternatives in the way of nutrition, home and body care. We are part of this healing revolution, by choosing to be proactive, live lovingly and see through open eyes.

When we choose to develop ourselves personally, we choose to facilitate the great change we collectively long to see in our world. We want to sparkle, and by embracing the magic of life with joy and gratitude, one by one we can illuminate our world.

Sigmund Freud wrote that it is impossible to overlook the extent to which civilisation is built upon a renunciation of instinct. By honouring our instinct and reconnecting with our inner wisdom, we may build a new kind of civilised life on earth. When we tend to the needs of our spirits with care and respect we nourish not only our personal but our collective wellness and the wellness of nature. We can share the important sparkle we cultivate within ourselves through self-care to bring joy, intuitive wisdom and comfort to each other and our world as we live.

Our light matters.

There is a wonderful Chinese proverb teaching that tension is who we think we should be while relaxation is who we are. Granting ourselves permission to settle into our true selves, to sparkle in tune with the calls of our wild and free spirits, is a revolutionary and necessary art. It could be said that much of the psychological suffering with which we are diagnosed in modern life is indeed spiritual suffering. A deep sense of loss of belonging; of unfilled desires of our spirits; of longing for a ritualistic, interconnected, magical and fulfilling way of life in connection with nature.

Indeed, we are starting to understand the significance of returning to nature now; to natural rhythms and what is authentic, organic, lasting and real. We are actively seeking ways to slow down, be mindful, relax and replenish ourselves. Having experienced the fleeting satisfaction of chasing things we don't actually need in pursuit of our happiness we are realising that we need to start new conversations around joy and meaning now.

Cracks are showing in the 'bigger, better, faster' model of living that has dominated our social and emotional landscapes for some time now. No matter how much we gather in the material world, including accolades, if we are forever rushed and feel disconnected from ourselves and our earth, we cannot find or enjoy our sparkle. In my eyes, the restlessness and separation that we have come to know in modern life is inviting a deeply meaningful and truly healing revolution.

In our fast-paced, demanding days we are now seeking relief, equanimity and liberation. We no longer want to feel fatigued, disillusioned, overworked and overwhelmed, distanced from the simple needs and pleasures that actually make us happy as human beings. We want to feel energised, inspired, soothed and nourished; to carry ourselves with a sense of our divinity, integrity and courage. We want to sparkle and we deserve to realise that, despite our layers of well-worn patterns, limiting beliefs and ideas, we were born to do so. Rather than spending our days feeling self-conscious, anxious and doubtful, we yearn to know and be our free, unbridled and true selves. We long to live daily lives enchanted by delicious spontaneity and profound delight. After all, we are not here to toil and suffer, we are here to know, touch and nurture heaven on earth.

We can begin to see and live
magically from this day forward.
We can stop searching and start finding.
Finding our bliss, balance and inner peace;
finding our sparkle.

Your own self-realisation
is the greatest service you
can render the world.

Ramana Maharshi

Journal Prompts

To me, bliss means . . .

In my eyes, the present moment is . . .

I feel happiest when . . .

I have noticed these messages from my spirit lately . . .

I am kindest to myself when . . .

In these ways, I can care more for myself . . .

In these ways, I can care more for others . . .

To me, work means . . .

I enjoy this kind of work . . .

I lose myself with pleasure when . . .

If I didn't have so many distractions I would spend more time . . .

I can notice these three particular details around me right now . . .

I can notice these three things within me right now . . .

I notice my breathing when . . .

I love my body when . . .

I appreciate my mind when . . .

My spirit is . . .

If my inner sparkle could talk . . .

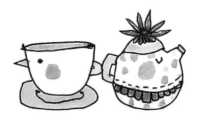

Affirmations

I AM FREE TO SOOTHE
AND COMFORT MYSELF

I AWAKEN DAILY
TO THE MAGIC OF LIFE

I CREATE BEAUTIFUL SPACES
WITHIN AND AROUND ME

I EXPRESS MY CREATIVITY WITH EASE

I ALLOW MYSELF TO EMBRACE JOY

I TAKE PLEASURE IN LEARNING
NEW THINGS

I AM ALWAYS LOVED, GUIDED
AND SUPPORTED

AMONGST NATURE I AM
FOREVER AT HOME

I AM POWERED BY LOVE

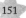

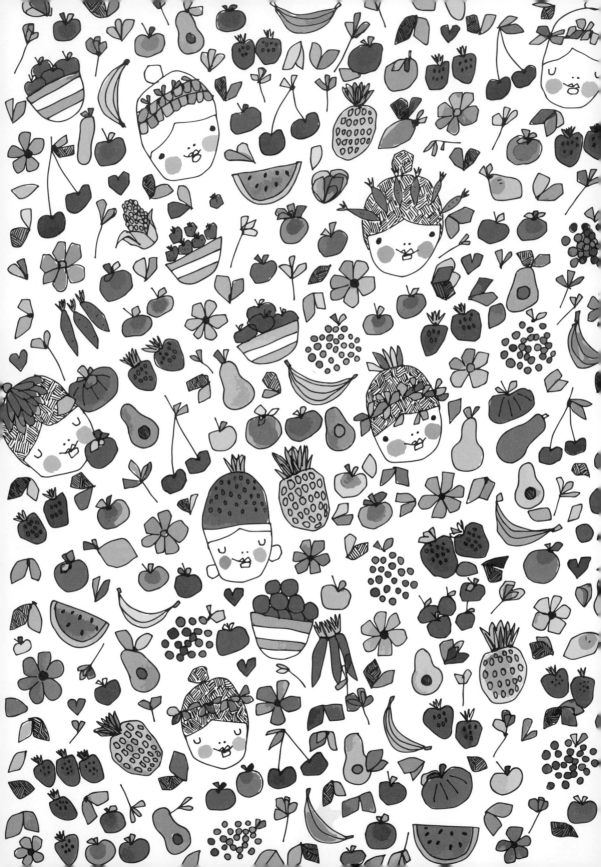

NOURISHING
YOUR SPARKLE

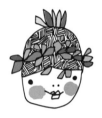

The lightness and joy of being in a magical world can be celebrated in all that we are and all that we do. This section offers daily inspiration for nourishing your spirit, exploring how making thoughtful choices in support of your sparkle can transform your experience of life.

Explore the healing powers of nature, the divine magic of whole foods from the earth, and the ways in which your environment and lifestyle shape your sparkle. Embrace the many exciting possibilities available to you as you choose to see life as precious, and experience the fullness of living. Nourish your spirit by celebrating your life with creativity, gratitude and magical awareness. Live all your moments in courageous, free expression of all that you are, and all that you can be.

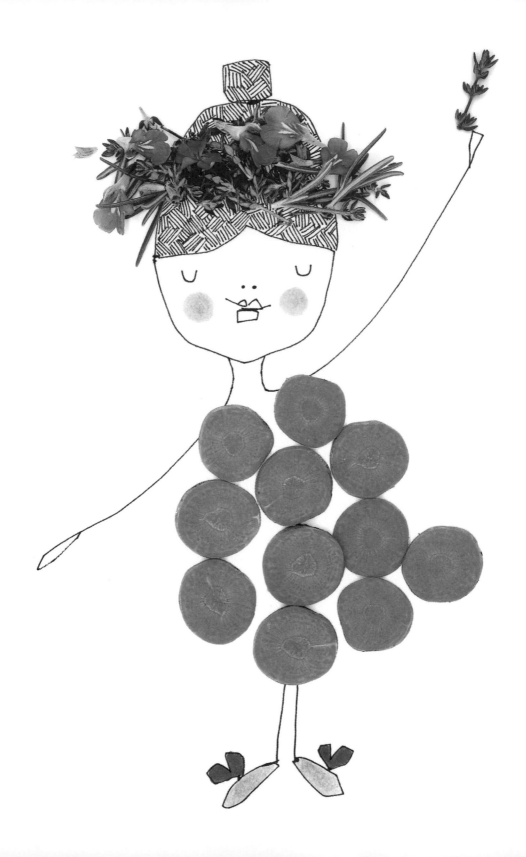

Nourishment for Life

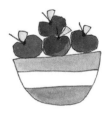

Nourishing our sparkles is a moment-to-moment pleasure. Decadent self and beauty care that connects and harmonises our minds, bodies and spirits is the ultimate kind of daily care. Rituals that unite and ground us are also essential ingredients for radiant wellbeing, bringing us comfort, inspiration and a sense of belonging. Natural whole foods brimming with life and energy from the earth and eaten with care become fuel for our spirits as much as our physical bodies and minds. Immersing ourselves in nature is deeply therapeutic and healing for us all. Indeed, with our love and attention, any and every day can become a tribute to our luminous, magical spirits.

William Blake wrote that what we call the body is a portion of our soul discerned by our five senses – the chief 'inlets' of our souls in this time and place. Indeed, it is through the sensory experiences of touching, hearing, seeing, smelling and tasting that we truly live; that we sense the life of our spirits, engaging, delighting in and expanding our sparkles. Rumi wrote that there are a thousand ways to kneel and kiss the ground, and a thousand ways to go home again. When he writes of 'home', in my eyes Rumi means back to our true selves, our innermost essence: our spirit. Indeed, there are so many ways to return to this place. Let us begin with the delight of eating, as this is something to which each one of us can relate.

Imagine eating a ripe, juicy peach with your full appreciation and attention. This luxury begins with noticing the divine colours on the skin of the peach, feeling its velvety skin and plumpness in your hands, tracing its curved edges with your fingers. It follows to taking the first bite into the peach with your teeth, tasting a sublime burst of sweetness, and the feeling of juice dripping down your chin and fingers. It involves the tiny seed from which the peach tree grew; the earth, fire, wind, water, sun and moon that created the earthly conditions in which the peach tree came to be and flourished; and the hands that picked the peach from its branch.

The gift of edible nourishment from nature is profound and immense. The hurried ways in which we eat, shop and live now thieve such an important piece of our joy. The joy of living. We too often eat mindlessly, sometimes even on the go. We can begrudgingly prepare meals, feeling strained and time-poor, use poor-quality ingredients and have no sense of connection to the earth, the farmer who cultivated the produce, or even the produce itself. Caring for our sparkles with edible nourishment involves not only choosing deeply nutritious, natural foods that heal and fortify us at a cellular level, it involves the acts of touching, choosing, preparing, serving and savouring food at the spiritual level. Ralph Waldo Emerson wrote that gluttony is never possible when we eat mindfully, but inevitable when we eat without care.

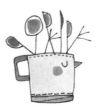

Another way to come 'home' is through nature therapy. While ideas around the therapeutic benefits of connecting with our earth were initially intuitive in nature, in recent years they have become scientifically proven to reduce stress, boost immunity and grow our joy. When we consider that stress is the greatest contributor to disease on our earth, and thus a tremendous burden for ourselves, our loved ones, and our health (or rather 'disease') care systems, we may fully grasp the need for us to truly relax and ground ourselves lovingly, mind, body and spirit.

In his book *Shinrin-yoku: The Japanese Way of Forest Bathing for Health and Relaxation*, Professor Yoshifumi Miyazaki writes that for eons, human beings have lived amongst nature. It is since the Industrial Revolution, only a couple of hundred years, that so many of us have become urbanised and profoundly affected by increasing technological stress. This means that for the overwhelming majority of human history on earth, we have lived within nature. The stress of modern life, incongruent with nature, her rhythms and wisdom, is causing radical increases in physical and mental health issues. It is no wonder that many human beings are permanently stressed; our human genes have not had long

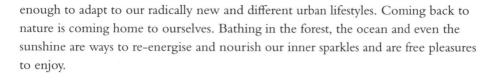

enough to adapt to our radically new and different urban lifestyles. Coming back to nature is coming home to ourselves. Bathing in the forest, the ocean and even the sunshine are ways to re-energise and nourish our inner sparkles and are free pleasures to enjoy.

Natural approaches to eating, drinking, looking after ourselves and the environments in which we live are ways that we can nourish our inner sparkles and refresh our spirits. We are fortified not only by the deliciousness of our attention to life, our self-care and self-love, but on a deeper level: as we love and respect our earth, we nurture and protect the roots of our real wellness. And not only our own wellness at that, but also the wellness of other beings and the future generations to roam this earth. We do not have a planet B; this is our earth. Our home. We are called to live in harmony with her, inspired by her, nourished, nurtured and held by her. We are being called to love, listen in and learn from her, sparkling together in unison.

It is devastating and unforgivable that in our human quest for more – our obsession with ownership and with our heavy treading upon her – our beautiful, bountiful earth is in deep pain. When our earth's sparkle is tarnished and extinguished, so is our own. We forge ahead, many of us oblivious to the truth that the sickness and suffering of our earth is our own sickness and suffering. Indeed, when our earth is stressed and diseased, so are we. The air we breathe, the water we drink, the soil in which we grow our food are our human foundations. When we pollute our waterways, cut down our trees, ransack and dirty our earth, contaminate our soils and stuff our earth's surface with our waste, our own spirits are angered and grieve too. We often wonder why we can feel so sad and disillusioned. It is because we are feeling with our earth.

We may not know quite where to begin healing our earth's sparkle. We may feel disheartened by the damage already done. Yet all the while, change begins with us. Finding new ways to embrace and love ourselves and our earth more is simply a matter of learning. In the lovely words of Mark Twain, 'Training is everything. The peach was once a bitter almond; cauliflower is nothing but cabbage with a college education!' Let us be the peaches and cauliflowers of our time and educate ourselves into a brighter, sparklier, happier and healthier future. Let us find ways to live within nature, humbly sharing our love with our earth, taking only that which we need, and embracing the magic and inspiration that nature effortlessly, generously offers us in all that we do.

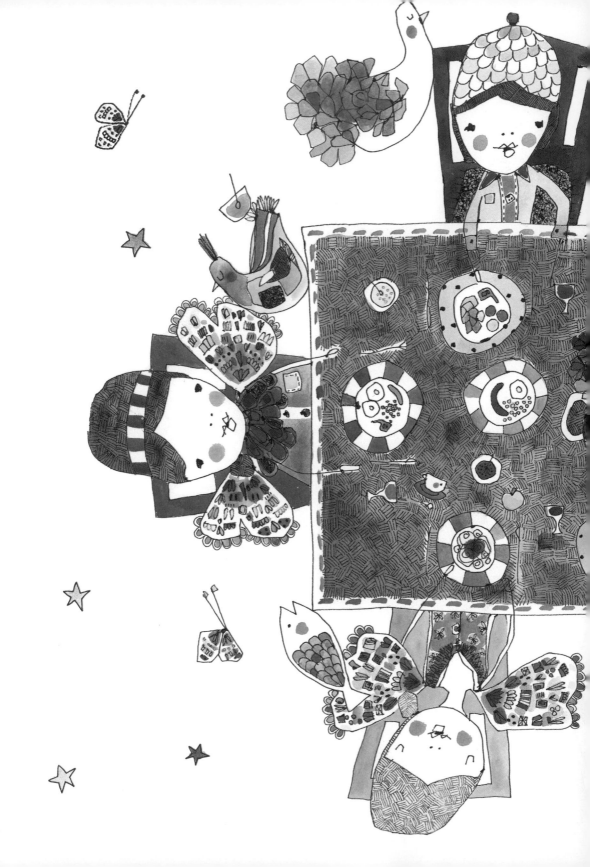

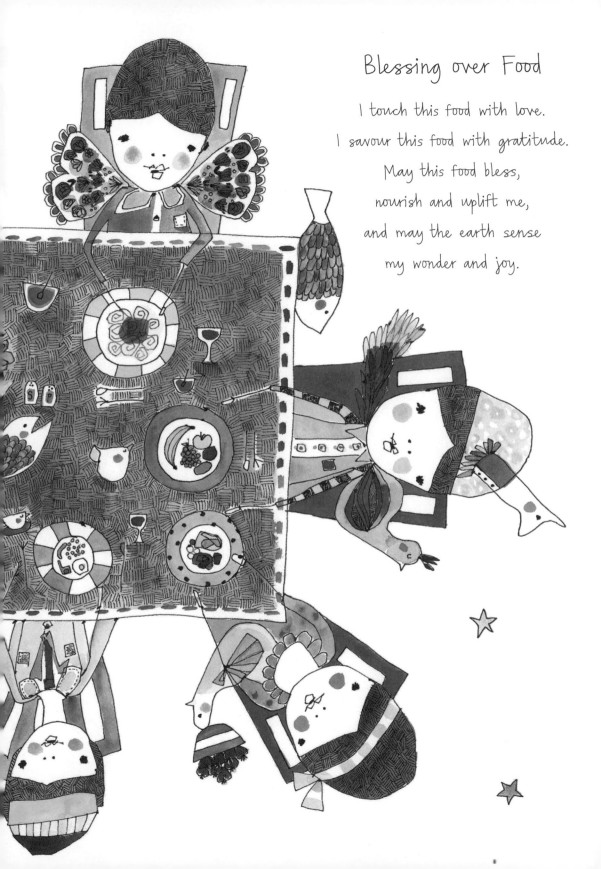

Blessing over Food

I touch this food with love.
I savour this food with gratitude.
May this food bless,
nourish and uplift me,
and may the earth sense
my wonder and joy.

SACRED NOURISHMENT

Real food is sacred. The world over, food is associated with pleasure
and joy, storytelling and connection, creative expression, love and care.
When we see food as precious and nourish our bodies in tune with nature,
our lives are transformed.

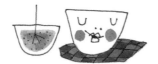

Experiencing the food we eat with gratitude and pleasure is a joy. William Shakespeare wrote ''Tis an ill cook that cannot lick his own fingers'! Getting messy in the kitchen, touching, feeling, creating with natural whole foods is an immersive, creative pleasure. The vast array of colourful fruits, vegetables, nuts, seeds, grasses and whole grains available to us provide limitless inspiration for creativity and indulgence. The natural colours in our foods convey their healing, fortifying and medicinal qualities. The more colourfully we eat, the greater variety of vitamins and minerals we take in to refresh our sparkles. Growing herbs in our gardens or on our windowsills, sprouting tiny seeds on our bench-tops, soaking nuts and whole grains and pickling delicious jars of vegetables are simple and joyous activities to explore and enjoy. If we can grow fruits and vegetables ourselves, or source them at a farm gate or farmers' market, we are blessed.

Clear, bright, sparkling eyes, luminous skin and a bountiful life force are outer markers of our inner sparkles, our bodies and spirits illuminated with sacred nourishment. Clear thinking, a joyous personal energy, peace of mind and a sense of connection, compassion and harmony with Mother Earth are sparkling, spiritual markers of true nourishment. When we embrace the magic of life and of our very own bodies we are naturally, inevitably compelled to make healthy choices in support of our wellness. We see no other alternative; it simply feels right to nourish ourselves in harmony with nature. We also see that delighting in food is nothing less than a spiritual experience.

The foods we eat can either grow or slow us. The food we eat not only fuels us for life and builds our bodies, it affects our moods, stress and energy levels, contributes to the balance or imbalance of our hormones, and shapes our gut and mental health. The quality of our food and the way we eat affects all aspects of our worlds, including our ability to concentrate and nurture relationships. It can determine our experiences of either deep healing or debilitating disease. Given that food is such a vital aspect of our wellbeing and moment-to-moment lives, we are wise to attend to the foods we choose to eat.

We are also wise to explore food as medicine. Healing foods are powerful elixirs for preventing and treating illness. Indeed, Mother Nature has a perfectly adequate, magical medicine cabinet fit to treat us all. Strengthening, cleansing and adaptogenic foods, herbs and natural remedies have been prescribed and taken since the dawn of time.

A healthy, happy and grateful spirit is the greatest tonic for our bodies and minds. It is a great tragedy when we associate edible nourishment with shame and guilt, expending our precious energy for life counting calories, worrying about what we eat, punishing, controlling and depriving ourselves through food. We cannot sparkle when we live this way. Common approaches to dieting and punishing exercise see many people regain the weight they once lost and feel deeply disappointed, disillusioned and unhappy. We need to listen in and nourish our sparkles on a deeper, more mindful level if we wish to experience truly radiant, sustainable wellbeing.

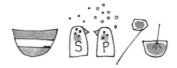

When we see our food as sacred and our bodies as worthy of real, whole food, we eat just as much as we need to be fulfilled and satisfied. We become attuned to our bodies and have a clear sense of their needs, likes and dislikes. We develop rituals and routines around the times of day we like to eat and the types of foods that best feed our sparkles. When nourished we are energised to move and enjoy our bodies, exercising with pleasure. We can begin to heal our confusion, stress and tension, making way for the truly joyous, intuitive relationship with our food and earth we deserve to know. Such a relationship is essential for our health and happiness.

Food is not only delicious and nourishing, it is a form of information for our bodies. The simpler and clearer the information, the easier it is for our bodies to understand and assimilate. Our natural bodies recognise natural foods; foods that support and rebuild us daily for life; foods that create healthy blood and bones, happy, healthy organs and sparkling cells. Chemicals, artificial colours, sweeteners, flavour enhancers and additives of all kinds in the processed foods we eat deplete and sicken us. They affect our minds and bodies in profound, unwanted ways. So much unnecessary disease and suffering can be prevented simply by transforming our ways with food. This is why for sparkling health and happiness I always choose natural, uncomplicated, nutrient-rich whole foods. I joyously draw on ingredients my eyes and my body can recognise. I enjoy celebrating these ingredients through simple cooking, and by savouring my food with great delight.

One of the most important lessons I have learned is to take care to eat light at night; it allows our bodies to detoxify overnight without the burden of digesting a heavy meal, is great for the management of our healthy weight, and allows us to wake up with far greater clarity and energy. I also activate all my nuts and seeds. This involves soaking them and slow-drying them in a very low-temperature oven; it makes them more digestible and removes any unwanted surface nasties. You can also buy them pre-activated at most good health food stores. Wherever possible I prefer to eat freshly prepared food rather than packaged, defrosted or reheated food. Fresh food fills our bodies with energising nutrients, uplifting us with rainbows of colour, and imbues us with real aliveness.

Hippocrates taught that all disease begins in the gut. Understanding so much more about the connection between the gut and brain as we do now through modern science, we can see that a suffering digestive system can have far-reaching and profound consequences. Depression, anxiety, brain fog, low mood, skin conditions and systematic inflammation are just several examples of suffering that can be related to our compromised gut health. Choosing to eat fresh, natural, seasonal, nutrient-dense plant-based foods rich in pre- and pro-biotics, minimising or at best avoiding exposure to food chemicals such as pesticides and herbicides and pharmaceutical drugs, and drinking ample fresh water every day are simple, conscious approaches to supporting our lifelong wellness. Indeed, high energy, radiant, dewy skin, bright eyes and agile, active bodies are outer markers of deep nourishment. To learn more about the link between gut health and your sparkle, please explore the 'Sparkling Resources' list on pages 226–228.

I have included a little collection of my favourite recipes for daily sparkling – basic plant-based recipes that I hope you will enjoy. Through these recipes I endeavour to show you how simple, rewarding and sacred food is. On page 159 you will find a lovely prayer to bless your food before enjoying it, plus a mindful eating meditation on pages 178–179.

Super Sparkles Smoothie

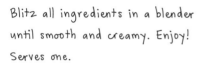

1 big handful of strawberries
2 big handfuls of baby spinach leaves
375 ml (12½ fl oz/1½ cups) plant mylk
  of choice
1 heaped tablespoon hemp seeds
4 brazil nuts
1 medjool date, pitted (optional)
pinch of cinnamon (optional)

Blitz all ingredients in a blender
until smooth and creamy. Enjoy!
Serves one.

Decadence Smoothie

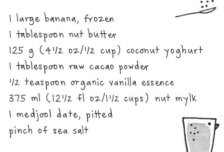

1 large banana, frozen
1 tablespoon nut butter
125 g (4½ oz/½ cup) coconut yoghurt
1 tablespoon raw cacao powder
½ teaspoon organic vanilla essence
375 ml (12½ fl oz/1½ cups) nut mylk
1 medjool date, pitted
pinch of sea salt

Blitz all ingredients in a blender
until smooth and creamy. Delicious!
Serves one.

Jupiter Juice

2 beetroot (beets), ends trimmed
3 cucumbers
1 big handful of kale
1 small knob of ginger

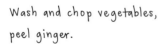

Wash and chop vegetables,
peel ginger.

Feed all ingredients through your
juicer and enjoy immediately!
Serves one or two.

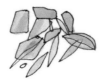

Green Fields Juice

½ bunch of celery
1 small fennel bulb
1 green apple
½ lemon, peeled
1 handful of baby spinach leaves
1 small handful of mint sprigs

Wash and chop vegetables, pick
mint leaves from their stems.

Feed all ingredients through your
juicer and enjoy immediately!
Serves one or two.

MATCHA GREEN SMOOTHIE

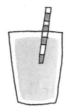

I will happily find any way to draw on the goodness of matcha green tea in my kitchen, not to mention smuggle in as many life-giving greens in my cooking as possible! Brimming with antioxidants and ready to boost your energy levels, matcha green tea is a wonderful offering from nature that takes this smoothie to the next level. It's a lovely way to start the day, an ideal post-workout drink or a wise 3 pm pick-me-up option. My plant mylk of choice is coconut, but feel free to use whichever you prefer. You can use a room-temperature banana if you don't have a frozen one on hand, but a frozen one, blitzed with a high-speed blender, will ensure a smooth and creamy finish. Serves one.

1 frozen banana, peeled and roughly chopped
375 ml (12½ fl oz/1½ cups) plant mylk of
  your choice
1 small handful of cashew nuts
1 small handful of kale leaves, torn
1 small handful of baby spinach leaves
½ teaspoon matcha green tea powder
1 medjool date, pitted
shredded coconut, to serve

Blitz all ingredients together in a high-speed blender and serve, topped with shredded coconut.

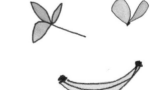

Soothing Hot Chocolate

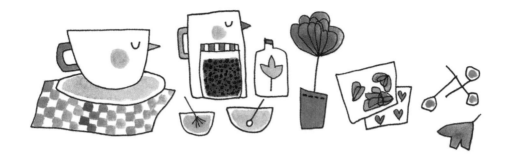

In my eyes this is one sacred recipe. Do not be scared of powdered medicinal mushrooms in your hot chocolate. They are an incredible source of extremely valuable, adaptogenic mind-body nutrients, and any taste they may have is disguised in this utterly dreamy, creamy, chocolatey blend. Hemp seeds offer us very impressive amounts of fibre, protein, potassium, vitamin A and iron. Enjoy in the morning for sustained energy, or in the evening as a soothing nightcap. Serves one.

375 ml (12½ fl oz/1½ cups) nut mylk, well warmed over heat
1 heaped tablespoon raw cacao powder
½ teaspoon reishi powder (or preferred mushroom mix)
½ teaspoon maca powder
1 heaped tablespoon hemp seeds
1 medjool date, pitted, or a dash of maple syrup
1 teaspoon tahini

Blend all ingredients together on high speed until thick and creamy. Enjoy wholeheartedly in your favourite mug.

Wild Rice with Chickpea Tempeh, Wilted Garlic Greens and Avocado Cream

This beautiful dish is so flavoursome and satisfying, combining nutrient-rich wild rice with life-giving dark leafy greens, protein-rich tempeh and the beautifying, body-loving goodness of avocado. Despite its name, wild rice is not a grain. It is the seed of a grass traditionally harvested in Canadian river beds and, among its other health benefits, it boasts sparkling levels of antioxidants and protein. Using garlic-infused oil and shallots, this dish ensures that it is fructose friendly without sacrificing any deliciousness whatsoever. Perfect for an easy lunch or dinner, or ideal savoured as a treat together with friends and loved ones. Serves four.

190 g (6½ oz/1 cup) wild rice,
  soaked overnight and rinsed
1 bay leaf
2 kaffir lime leaves
2 tablespoons garlic-infused oil
300 g (10½ oz) chickpea tempeh, crumbled
250 g (9 oz) mixed dark leafy greens
  (spinach, kale, silverbeet etc)
1 handful of roughly chopped spring onions
  (scallions), green part only
2 tablespoons tamari
1 tablespoon mirin
1 big handful of baby sprouts to garnish
30 g (1 oz/¼ cup) pepitas (pumpkin seeds),
  toasted, to garnish

AVOCADO CREAM

2 avocados
90 g (3 oz/⅓ cup) coconut yoghurt
2 tablespoons of lemon or lime juice
pinch of chilli flakes
dash of mirin

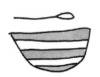

Avocado cream is perfect on crunchy sourdough toast too, piled high with fresh leafy greens

Place wild rice in a saucepan with 750 ml (25½ fl oz/ 3 cups) of filtered water, the bay leaf and kaffir lime leaves. Bring to the boil then reduce the heat, simmering for 20–30 minutes until you notice the rice puffing open in white curls that are tender upon taste-testing. Once ready, turn off the heat, strain any excess water, return to the saucepan and put the lid on.

While the rice is cooking, blitz all the avocado cream ingredients in a small food processor until very smooth. Season to taste with freshly ground black pepper and sea salt, adding more chilli flakes to taste if desired.

Once the wild rice is almost done, warm the garlic-infused oil over medium heat in a heavy-based frying pan. Add the crumbled tempeh, tossing until just browned. Add the greens, spring onions, tamari and mirin, stirring well to coat. Stir over medium heat until the greens are wilted. Add your tempeh and greens to your wild rice, stirring well to combine.

Serve in your favourite bowls and top with dollops of avocado cream, garnishing with the baby sprouts and toasted pepitas.

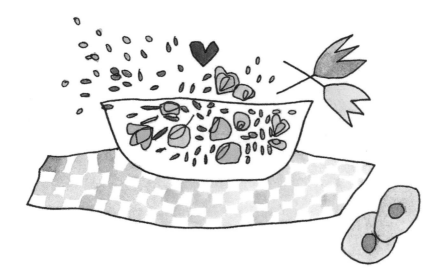

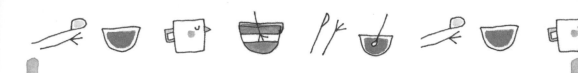

HEALING SOUP

When in need of comfort and healing, I always turn to this
beautiful, simple soup. Miso makes a nourishing, flavoursome
broth, and a lovely base for all the fortifying vegetables and
herbs. It's a lovely light evening meal, or a restorative bowl
of goodness when in need of some healing. If you would like
a little extra sustenance, add a scoop of steamed basmati rice
to each bowl before serving. Serves four.

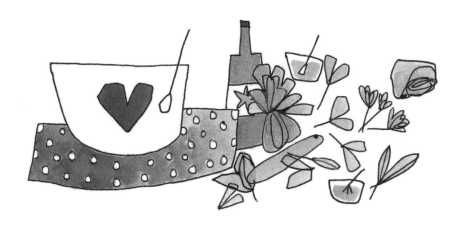

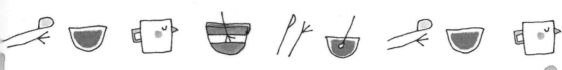

SOUP

2 tablespoons garlic-infused oil
3 carrots, finely chopped
3 zucchini (courgettes), finely chopped
1 large tomato, diced
1 small knob of ginger, minced
3 tablespoons miso paste
2 tablespoons tamari
2 tablespoons mirin
2 kaffir lime leaves
1 bay leaf
1 small bunch (3 stems) bok choy
   (pak choy), thinly sliced
1 big handful of spinach leaves
1 big handful of rainbow chard or
   kale leaves, torn
1 handful of finely chopped spring onions
   (scallions), green part only
1 cup cooked basmati rice (optional)
pinch of chilli flakes (optional)

GARNISH

coriander leaves (cilantro)
fresh lemon or lime juice
drizzle of tamari (optional)
1 tablespoon nutritional yeast flakes
   (optional)

Set a big heavy-based saucepan over
medium heat and gently warm the
garlic-infused oil. Add the carrots,
zucchini, tomato, ginger, miso, tamari,
mirin, lime leaves and bay leaf and
stir gently for a few minutes.

Add 1.25 litres (42 fl oz/ 5 cups)
of filtered water and bring to the
boil. Reduce the heat and simmer
for 10 minutes.

Add the bok choy, spinach and rainbow
chard or kale leaves and spring onions
and cook lightly for another few
minutes. If seeking more broth, add
more filtered water and simmer gently
for another 10 minutes. Remove from
the heat.

If using rice, place a scoop of steamed
basmati rice in the bottom of each bowl
then ladle the soup over.

Top the soup with coriander leaves,
fresh lemon or lime juice, and a drizzle
of tamari, if desired. For an extra dose
of vitamin B and a nutty, cheesy flavour,
sprinkle with nutritional yeast flakes.

Roasted Rainbow Vegetables with Caramelised Hazelnuts and Dreamy Creamy Dressing

I love the colour and comfort roasted vegetables deliver, and savour the different varieties seasonally throughout the year. Draw on whatever vegetables you have on hand, or follow the recipe below. Garnish with greens and caramelised hazelnuts for added texture and goodness. Drizzle with dreamy dressing to add even more magic! Serves four to six.

900 g (2 lbs/1/4 large) kent pumpkin (winter squash), roughly chopped
650 g (1½ lb) sweet potatoes, skin on and roughly chopped
2 carrots, roughly chopped
650 g (1½ lb) Dutch cream potatoes, skin on and roughly chopped
2 zucchini (courgettes), roughly chopped
1 red capsicum (bell pepper), roughly chopped
2 tablespoons extra-virgin olive oil
1 teaspoon dried thyme leaves
1 teaspoon sweet paprika (optional)
1 handful of spring onions (scallions), green part only, finely chopped, to garnish
2 handfuls of wild rocket (arugula), to garnish

CARAMELISED HAZELNUTS

125 g (4½ oz/1 cup) hazelnuts
2 tablespoons tamari
2 tablespoons maple syrup
a crack of freshly ground black pepper
pinch of salt
pinch of chilli flakes (optional)

CREAMY DRESSING

185 g (6¾ oz/3/4 cup) coconut yoghurt
1 tablespoon garlic-infused oil
2 teaspoons wholegrain mustard
2 tablespoons mirin
2 teaspoons tahini
2 tablespoons fresh lemon juice
1 small handful of freshly cut chives
pinch of chilli flakes (optional)

Preheat the oven to 200°C (400°F). Lay the chopped vegetables evenly on a baking tray. Drizzle with the olive oil, sprinkle with salt, pepper, thyme, and sweet paprika, if desired. Bake for 40 minutes or until the vegetables are crispy outside, soft inside.

Meanwhile, blitz all the dressing ingredients together until smooth and creamy. Whisk through with small splashes of filtered water until your desired consistency is reached. Season with freshly ground black pepper and sea salt to taste.

To make the caramelised hazelnuts, set a frying pan over high heat. Add the hazelnuts, tamari and maple syrup, stirring, until caramelised. Season with the pepper, salt and chilli flakes, if desired. Set aside on baking paper to cool.

Arrange the baked vegetables thoughtfully on your favourite serving platter. Drizzle liberally with the creamy dressing and sprinkle with the finely chopped spring onion, the rocket and caramelised hazelnuts to finish.

Use your dressing immediately or store in an airtight container in the fridge for up to 4 days. Just whisk and add a little more water before enjoying any leftover dressing you might have.

HAPPINESS SALAD WITH CRISPY TOFU BITES

This colourful salad is delicious, nourishing and enlivening, with a delectable mix of flavours and textures sure to delight! I always choose organic or biodynamic tofu, and appreciate the pressed variety for its extra firmness. This salad is perfect for picnics as it travels very well. Simply pack the dressing separately, and toss it through just before serving. This salad serves four, happily.

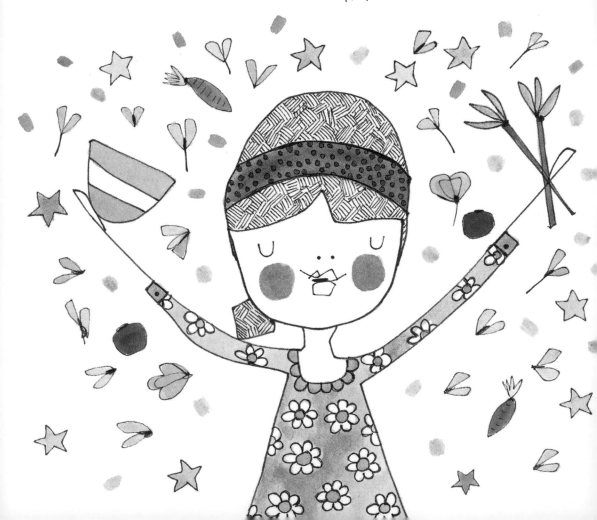

4 big handfuls of mixed leafy greens,
  e.g. wild rocket (arugula), baby spinach
  leaves and sprouts
2 carrots, coarsely grated
2 medium beetroot (beets), grated
180 g (6 oz/1 cup) black kalamata olives, pitted
1 ripe avocado, sliced
1 handful of shredded coconut, to garnish
1 big handful of coriander (cilantro) sprigs,
  to garnish
50 g (1³/4 oz/¹/3 cup) toasted sesame seeds,
  to garnish

CRISPY TOFU BITES
350 g (12½ oz) organic tofu, cubed
1 tablespoon coconut oil, melted
2 tablespoons tamari
1 tablespoon mirin
2 teaspoons sesame oil
1 garlic clove, minced
1 teaspoon paprika
1 teaspoon smoked paprika
1 teaspoon ground cumin
1 teaspoon ground turmeric
1 tablespoon apple cider vinegar

SALAD DRESSING
3 tablespoons tamari
1 tablespoon mirin
2 tablespoons extra-virgin olive oil
1 tablespoon maple syrup
2 teaspoons mustard
juice of ½ a lime
dash of filtered water

To make the tofu bites, place the cubed tofu in a mixing bowl. Add the remaining ingredients, stir and let it marinate for 10 minutes.

Meanwhile, whisk the salad dressing ingredients together and season to taste with sea salt and freshly ground black pepper. Set aside.

Toss the marinated tofu bites in a hot wok or frying pan and stir over medium heat until cooked through and crisp (about 7–10 minutes). If the wok dries out, add little splashes of water to avoid sticking. Once it's ready, set aside.

Assemble your green leaves, grated carrot and beetroot, olives and sliced avocado on your favourite serving plates. Add the crispy tofu bites and drizzle joyously with the dressing. Garnish with the shredded coconut, coriander and sesame seeds, serve and savour!

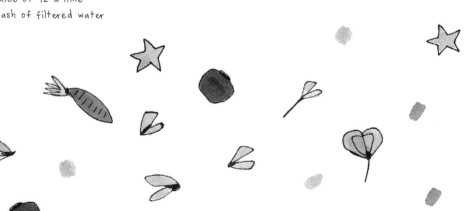

RAW CARAMEL SLICE

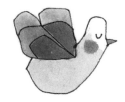

This must be one of my most requested recipes when it comes to sharing with friends and loved ones! Don't be put off by its three parts; they are so easy to make and a joy to assemble. This slice is so finger-licking delicious and nutrient dense and, when cut into smaller squares, makes for perfect snacking. Young and more grown-up hearts alike will relish this recipe because it's a little slice of heaven.

While it's nearly impossible, I urge you to exercise restraint and wait until this slice fully sets before cutting it. You may of course lick the spatula after making your caramel – something I highly recommend! By waiting for this slice to set fully you will ensure neat, firm pieces that are easy to handle, serve and share.

This slice will keep in an airtight container in the freezer for weeks. Simply defrost it for 20–30 minutes prior to serving and serve either chilled or at room temperature for ultimate enjoyment. In the spirit of wasting nothing at all, I add 500 ml (17 fl oz/2 cups) of filtered water to the blender after scooping the caramel out, making a little salted caramel mylkshake to knock my own socks off! Makes 24 good squares.

BASE

140 g (5 oz/1 cup) mixed raw
  unsalted nuts
90 g (6 oz/1½ cup) buckinis (activated
  buckwheat groats)
45 g (1½ oz/½ cup) desiccated
  (shredded) coconut
2½ tablespoons coconut oil
80 ml (2½ fl oz/⅓ cup) maple syrup
pinch of salt

CARAMEL

16 dates, pitted and soaked in warm
  water for at least 15 minutes
270 g (9½ oz/1 cup) tahini
pinch of salt
400 ml (13½ fl oz) additive-free
  coconut cream

CHOCOLATE

60 g (2 oz/½ cup) raw cacao powder
80 ml (2½ fl oz/⅓ cup) maple syrup
1 teaspoon organic vanilla essence
80 ml (2½ fl oz/⅓ cup) coconut oil

Blitz the base ingredients in a food processor. Press into the base of a glass or ceramic dish measuring approximately 30 cm × 40 cm (12 in × 16 in). Chill in the freezer while you prepare the other elements.

For the caramel, blitz the ingredients until creamy and smooth. Pour the caramel evenly atop the base and return to the freezer for at least 30 minutes.

In a medium saucepan, melt the chocolate ingredients together over low heat, adding up to 60 ml (2 fl oz/¼ cup) room-temperature water until the sauce is smooth and glossy. Pour over the cooled caramel and return to the freezer for at least 4 hours to set, or until nice and firm and ready to slice. Enjoy with a cup of tea and a sparkle within!

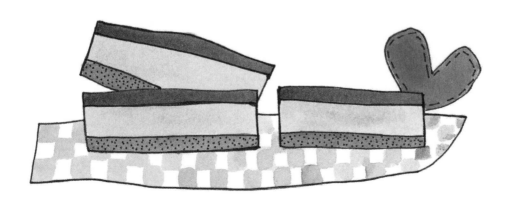

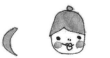

CHOC-MISO BLISS BALLS

These protein-rich, flavoursome chocolate bliss balls never last long in our little nest. With the surprisingly delicious, healthful addition of miso paste, these bliss balls pack a flavour punch that's hard not to love! Simply mix, roll and enjoy. Store in an airtight container for up to two weeks, and savour at your whim as nourishing little sweet treats. Makes 30 bliss balls.

225 g (8 oz/2½ cups) desiccated
  (shredded) coconut
85 g (3 oz/⅔ cup) raw cacao powder
180 g (6½ oz/⅔ cup) tahini
125 ml (4 fl oz/½ cup) maple syrup
1½ teaspoons organic vanilla essence
2 tablespoons coconut oil
140 g (5 oz/1 cup) mixed nuts
  (walnuts, cashews, Brazil nuts)
pinch of salt
1 heaped tablespoon miso paste
  (I use brown rice miso)
90 g (6 oz/1½ cup) buckinis
  (activated buckwheat groats)

Pulse 135 g (5 oz/1½ cups) of the coconut along with all the other ingredients, except the buckinis, in a food processor until clumps begin to form. Add tiny splashes of water if your mix feels at all dry.

Add the buckinis and stir gently to combine, keeping them crunchy and intact.

Using your hands, have fun rolling the mix into little balls, coating with the remaining desiccated coconut to finish.

Raspberry-Studded Lemon, Lime and Coconut Biscuits

These simple, moist and totally exquisite biscuits are favourites at home and a hit with friends! They are so satisfying and look very beautiful too. Perfect morning or afternoon tea treats, great for lunchboxes, and heavenly accompanied by a little tea ceremony. Makes 24 biscuits.

200 g (7 oz/ 2 cups) almond meal

65 g (2¼ oz/¾ cup) desiccated (shredded) coconut

2 tablespoons tapioca or arrowroot flour

60 ml (2 fl oz/¼ cup) coconut oil, melted and cooled

1 teaspoon organic vanilla essence

1 teaspoon organic food-grade lemon essential oil

1 tablespoon fresh lemon juice

1 teaspoon lemon zest

1 tablespoon fresh lime juice

1 teaspoon lime zest

60 ml (2 fl oz/¼ cup) maple syrup

pinch of sea salt

95 g (3½ oz/¾ cup) frozen organic raspberries

Preheat the oven to 175°C (350°F) and line a baking tray with baking paper. In a medium bowl, mix together all the ingredients, except the raspberries, until well combined. Using your hands, roll the mixture into little balls and place on the prepared baking tray.

Gently press a raspberry into the top of each biscuit, smoothing any cracked edges with your fingers.

Bake for 10–15 minutes, or until the biscuits are lightly golden underneath. They should still look and feel soft, but they will firm up when cooled.

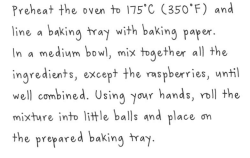

Mindful Eating Meditation

As I prepare to eat this food,
I take a few deep breaths.
Breathing in and breathing out,
I let all the hurries and worries of my day go,
and I relax.
Relaxing my mind and body now,
I bring myself back to this moment.
This is the only moment
and the most important moment
in my life right now.

Breathing in, I admire the food I see before me.
I notice colours and shapes,
textures and aromas,
and any memories conjured.
I thank this food for nourishing my body,
and I thank the earth for her riches.

I acknowledge the elements:
earth, wind, fire, air, water and ether
that make nourishment possible for me.
Elements without which I, and this food, would not exist.
With gratitude, I sense the immensity of my blessings now.

As I take my first mouthful of food,
I take the time to notice how it feels.
Chewing very slowly, I notice the flavours released upon my tongue:
sweetness, saltiness, sourness, bitterness.
I notice the flavours come to me.
I notice if they come all at once, or one after another.

Breathing deeply in and out, I notice the textures at play.
Is this food soft or crisp, crunchy, heavy or light?
I notice how my body feels about eating this particular food.
I let my mind and body speak to me as I go along.
As I eat on, I continue to breathe and smile. I take my time.

As I take in my food, I bless my body.
I thank my digestive system and see it smiling with joy.
I thank my body for looking after me every day,
I thank my food for building and sustaining me, moment to moment.
I see myself radiant, vital and brimming with sparkling energy.

When I am finished eating, I close my eyes and pause for a moment.
I savour my experience to the fullest.
When I feel ready I open my eyes and resume my day,
fulfilled and deeply nourished.

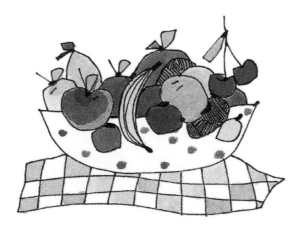

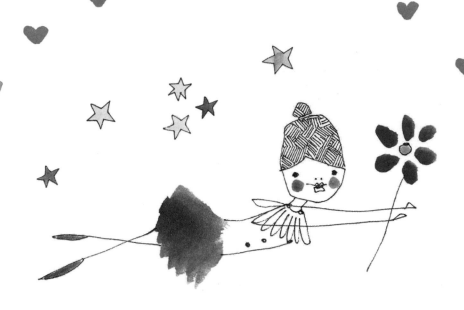

DEAR BODY,

THANK YOU.

I LOVE YOU.

M

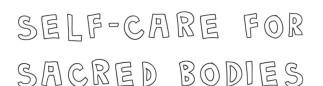

SELF-CARE FOR SACRED BODIES

When we love and honour ourselves we cannot help but sparkle.
We glow from within, luminous with peace of mind and spirit.
While our bodies look infinitely different on the outside, we all
share the same essential needs. To love ourselves deeply is
to find all that we have been looking for.

The pervasive visual culture in which we live today has resulted in our beautiful bodies being subjected to endless scrutiny and comparison. Our marvellous bodies, designed to carry us through life, were never meant to be treated in this way. Our pain is shared, as so many of us have lost our way when it comes to valuing, appreciating and really knowing our bodies. Re-establishing loving connection with our bodies is true healing. When we touch, praise and delight our bodies with our love, we cultivate the true joy and inner peace we seek.

Through daily self-care we nurture our wellness. We might enjoy mindful movement such as stretching exercises or yoga to nourish our mind–body bliss, showing us the many things our bodies are capable of doing and feeling. While fancy spa treatments are real luxuries, it is also possible to achieve moments of luxurious relaxation at home through simple self-care practices. We might enjoy a long, healing Epsom salt bath to soothe our weary muscles and refresh our skin, or indulgent little spa treatments such as self-massage, exfoliation or luscious moisturising to bring ourselves that sense of decadence we seek.

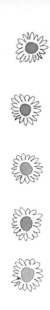

For beautiful skin, hair and teeth, healthy figures and a sparkling glow, we need look no further than natural beauty care. This beauty care starts within, with what we put into our bodies as edible nourishment. It also includes the way we treat our outer bodies with beauty products, make-up, skin- and hair-care. There are always natural alternatives for harmful products we might currently be using — alternatives that contribute to sustainable natural beauty and graceful ageing.

We may draw on very simple offerings from nature such as coconut oil, sea salt, apple cider vinegar and organic essential oils to create our own basic but decadent body-care products, and look into reputable natural brands that guarantee cruelty-free, organic make-up and body-care offerings. Check all labels very carefully as many beauty products, from deodorants to toothpastes, can contain hidden nasties. If you cannot read or understand what an ingredient is, know that your body will be baffled too. Let natural beauty-care rituals infuse your days with pleasure and joy, delighting your sparkling spirit.

To follow I have included a little collection of my personal favourite body-care recipes and rituals for daily radiance: simple ideas that I hope you will enjoy. With these inspirations I hope to show you how easy, healing and decadent natural body care is to enjoy. On pages 194–195 you will find a lovely prayer to bless your sacred body before or during your self-care exercises.

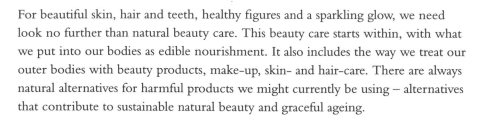

Beauty is the virtue of the body as virtue is the beauty of the soul.

Ralph Waldo Emerson

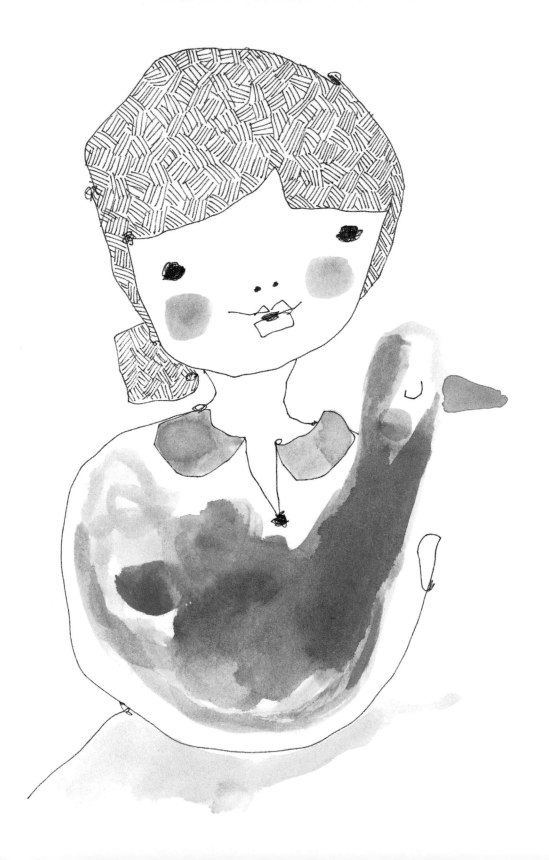

NATURAL BODY-CARE FOR SPARKLING

The magic and beauty of body-care rituals is that they not only help us to look and feel our sparkliest selves – they also harmonise our minds, bodies and spirits. Through the time and attention we give our bodies, we embrace ourselves with loving tenderness. This loving tenderness is more powerful than we realise: it is foundational for growing and nurturing the lifelong romance we are invited to cultivate with ourselves.

When we connect with our bodies we can lovingly call all parts of ourselves home to wholeness, grounding our minds and bodies in the present moment. Through our self-care rituals we express respect and gratitude for ourselves and our lives. Our wise, magnificent bodies carry us through life each day and do so many miraculous things. We often focus on what our bodies look like, but as magical homes for our luminous spirits, our bodies are so much more.

Oil pulling is one of my favourite daily rituals. I simply place a tablespoon of coconut oil in my mouth upon waking each morning and 'swoosh' it around for ten to twenty minutes. Not only does this contribute to optimum oral hygiene and a sparkly smile, Aryuvedic wisdom suggests that the ancient ritual of oil pulling may also assist to support our general wellness in curious and exciting ways. Begin by trying oil pulling for just a few minutes, and increase your swoosh time as you feel comfortable to. Another beautiful, Ayurvedic-inspired ritual is self-message with warmed oil. This exercise is featured on page 190. Self-massage is a deeply sacred and healing practice that helps us to cultivate more positive, tender relationships with our bodies. Dry body brushing and tongue cleaning are detoxifying, clarifying daily rituals to explore and enjoy, while organic face masks, body-care treatments and aromatherepeutic baths make for ultimate little luxuries. Savouring early nights, drinking ample fresh water and enjoying whole foods that nourish us deeply from within are tried and tested beauty remedies for daily sparkling.

As you move through these pages and inspirations, may you feel energised to explore natural beauty care in a new and refreshing way.

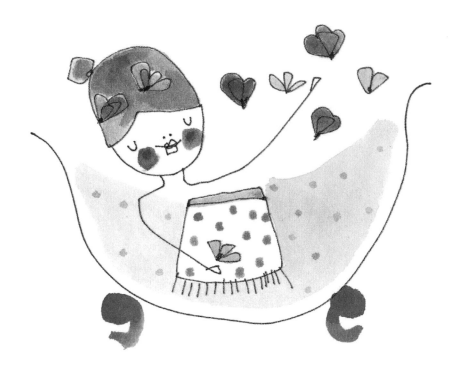

BODY-CARE RECIPES

Making our own natural body-care blends is a joyous pleasure. It is cost effective, fun and therapeutic for our bodies, minds and spirits. A simple collection of favourite organic essential oils, a little filtered water, coconut oil, sea salt, rose petals and kitchen pantry basics can go a very long way!

In order to make these inspirations as easy and appealing as possible, I have kept each recipe very simple. You will notice that the essential oil selections in each recipe are intentionally open. The beauty of exploring these body-care recipes is personalising fragrances that appeal to you, and experimenting with different scents to discover what ratios and varieties ignite or soothe your spirit. We are each intuitively drawn to different scents, often corresponding with the inherently healing and balancing qualities of the essential oils themselves. Explore your creativity and gather new wisdom, learning more about essential oils and their unique, remedial properties.

Scented Body Mists

Soothe and uplift yourself every day with beautiful homemade body mists. Many standard perfumes contain unwanted nasties that can disrupt our hormones, skin and sinuses and our sparkles. Drawing on organic essential oils, filtered water and, if we desire, a few little crystals for extra magic, we can create beautiful, safe body mists that smell and feel wonderful. I keep various therapeutic scents on hand each day, some to stimulate energy, others to invite rest and relaxation. Here are three simple and beautiful recipes for you to explore. May they inspire you to create your very own personalised blends with the scents you most love.

Love: 5 drops of geranium, 5 drops of grapefruit, 10 drops of sandalwood

Nourish: 10 drops of lavender, 5 drops of peppermint

Adventure: 3 drops of patchouli, 5 drops of primrose, 10 drops of sandalwood

Add the organic essential oils for your chosen recipe to a spray bottle with 100 ml (3½ fl oz) filtered water.

Add any little crystals of your choice.

Shake well, spritz and enjoy liberally.

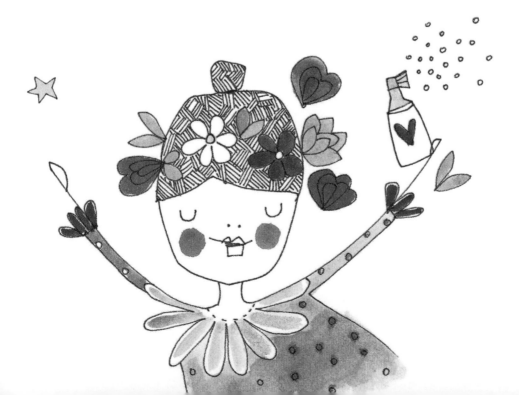

Coconut & Citrus Bath Melts

These simple bath melts take just minutes to make but allow for hours of bathing pleasure! A silicone ice-cube tray works wonders as its flexibility makes for the greatest ease of handling. You might even find an ice-cube tray that allows you to make love heart-, flower- or star-shaped bath melts for extra delight! The addition of fresh citrus zest in this recipe works beautifully with the decadent, luscious creaminess of coconut oil.

2 cups of unrefined organic coconut oil
2 tablespoons of citrus zest (lemon, lime, orange)
10 drops of geranium essential oil

Melt the coconut oil in a small saucepan, then allow to cool. Add the essential oil and citrus zest, then pour the mixture into your ice-cube tray and set in the freezer for 1-2 hours. Store them in the freezer until ready to use.

Enjoy a couple of melts per bath for a fragrant, moisturising and luxurious bathing experience.

Sparkle Scrub

The gentle exfoliating quality of this delightful, fragrant scrub makes it ideal for treating tired feet or reviving lacklustre, dry skin. Be sure to patch-test in advance to ensure that your skin approves of your blend.

1 cup coconut sugar
1/2 cup almond oil
1 teaspoon organic vanilla essence
15 drops of organic lavender essential oil

Simply mix all the ingredients together until well combined, and store in a small, airtight container.

To enjoy, massage the scrub gently into the skin. Rinse well, then moisturise with coconut oil, gently towel-drying excess oil.

Floral Bath Salts

Epsom salts have long been used for soothing sore, tired muscles and for detoxifying, grounding and nurturing the body. I love including spray-free rose petals in my bath salts for a touch of fragrance, colour and romance. Lavender, chamomile or jasmine petals also work beautifully. For an extra heavenly experience, simply add one full tin of coconut cream to your bath along with these pretty, healing salts. Enjoy.

4 cups epsom salts
20 drops wild rose
  essential oil
1 handful of spray-free petals

Mix all the ingredients together very well, then pour into an airtight glass jar.

To use, pour 1/2–1 cup of salts into your bath as it fills, then delight in a beautiful, soothing bathing experience.

Coconut & Aloe Vera Face Mask

Face masks are relaxing and fun to enjoy while being decadently, deeply nourishing for our skin. This simple, gentle recipe contains just two ingredients and works wonders even for very sensitive skin. As with all skin treatments, be sure to patch-test for suitability. If lying down to enjoy this mask, gently place cucumber slices over your eyes to help protect and soothe them.

3 tablespoons
  coconut yoghurt
1 teaspoon aloe vera gel
2 cucumber slices

Combine the coconut yoghurt and aloe vera gel and enjoy it immediately by spreading it gently and evenly over your face, being careful to avoid your delicate eye area. Leave it on for 10 minutes before rinsing well and moisturising with a little coconut oil or natural moisturiser of your choice.

SELF-MASSAGE FOR SPARKLING

There is a Ayurvedic-inspired little luxury that I love, and believe is most underrated: self-massage. In my eyes, this ritual is nothing short of magical. Over time it has helped me to connect with my body and learn to love my body as it truly deserves to be loved. We can spend a lot of time dishonouring our bodies. The immediacy, tenderness and directness of self-massage is profoundly healing.

Simply warm a little sesame or coconut oil in a saucepan and allow it to cool slightly. Lay a towel on your bathroom floor, take your clothes off, tie your hair up, and make yourself as comfortable as possible. You might like to light a candle, listen to some beautiful music or arrange some flowers in your space to make this ritual feel all the more special. During cooler months, make sure to warm your space for ultimate comfort.

When you are ready, begin massaging your body gently from the soles of your feet up to your neck and scalp, and even through your hair if desired. You can cleanse your hands then massage your face as well. Take as long as you please to enjoy these moments with your body. Make time for yourself. This massage is like a meditation and is true nourishment for your spirit. When you have finished, close your eyes for a moment. You might wish to offer your body a little prayer of love and gratitude. You have just gifted yourself with your love. Honour yourself now.

Following your massage and before hopping into a warm bath or bed, rinse off gently under the shower. This ritual may also be enjoyed in the morning before showering to begin the day on a completely different, healing and nurturing note. It also pairs beautifully with the Body Love Meditation on pages 194–195. I truly hope you will fall in love with this precious ritual, just as I have.

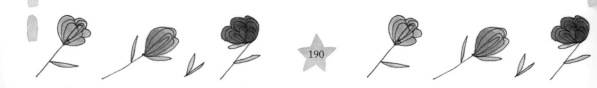

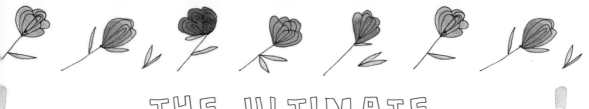

THE ULTIMATE BEAUTY THERAPIST

Walking down the beauty aisle of any store we are bombarded by products that promise to enhance our sparkle. The compelling truth is that the greatest secret to looking and feeling beautiful cannot be found on a shelf. It doesn't cost a cent, and it cannot be bought. The greatest secret to looking and feeling beautiful is our very own self-talk. A kind inner voice is the ultimate beauty therapist.

The opinions we hold of ourselves determine our inner dialogue, and our inner dialogue determines how we feel. When we approve of ourselves and know that we sparkle by design; that we are inherently beautiful, our very own kind of beautiful, we free ourselves to see beauty through new eyes, and experience it in radically new ways. Indeed, beauty that emanates from spirit level is beauty that bedazzles.

You are beautiful. Next time you doubt it, consider that you are made of stardust. Consider that you contain all the mysteries of the universe within you. Consider that you are enchanting and luminous just by being alive. In touch with our spirits we are forces of nature; we know ourselves to be utterly magical and completely divine.

Talk to yourself kindly, always. Talk to yourself with compassion and kindness on good and bad days, while looking in the mirror, while walking down the street, when alone and in the company of others. Intercept thoughts that hurt and limit you. Choose thoughts that support and uplift you. Let your inner voice be the kindest voice you know and approve of yourself, because your happiness depends on it.

This simple, free and powerful kind of beauty therapy may be different to what you have been sold in the past, but I urge you to embrace it from this day forward. Nurture, love and enjoy your inner voice, and discover the best beauty therapist of all time.

True beauty
flourishes with
more tenderness
more care
more grace
more kindness
more slow moments
more appreciation
more respect
more honesty
more courage
more faith

M

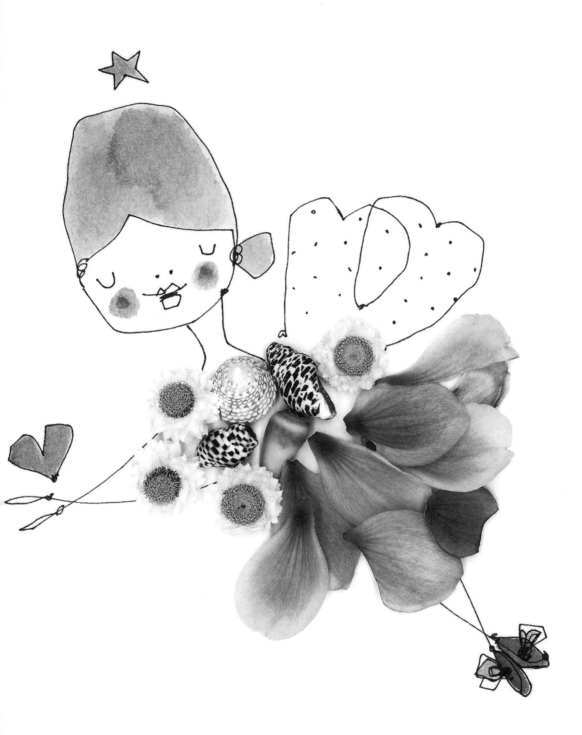

Body Love Meditation

Finding myself the most comfortable position
either sitting or lying down now,
I close my eyes and deepen my breathing.
Breathing in, and breathing out.

As I inhale, I feel energy rising up from deep within my belly,
right up through my chest, shoulders and neck,
circulating around my jaw and my eyes,
and moving up and out through the crown of my head.

Exhaling now, I breathe new light and air down,
right back through the top of my head and down into my body,
moving through my whole body, right down and out through the soles of my feet,
touching every edge, every cell.
I let my breath flow on in this way for a few more moments,
feeling gently aware of my whole body breathing.

I take this moment to talk to any parts of myself
that need special love.
Any parts that may be tight or strained,
gripping, tensing or feeling unloved.
I spend a few moments listening to these parts of me now,
breathing into them with care.
I ask them to accept my love,
and my efforts to love myself that little bit more,
each and every day.
Breathing in and out, I let healing energy fill my body,
nurturing me, nourishing me.

In this peaceful and quiet space
I offer myself forgiveness
for any hurtful thoughts or comments
I have made about my beautiful body.

For all the times I have abandoned myself.
Breathing in deeply now, I wholly forgive myself.
Breathing out, I deeply forgive my body.
In the release and tenderness of my forgiveness
I let myself feel all my feelings.
One breath at a time, deeply in and deeply out.

Breathing on, I see myself healthy, happy and fulfilled.
I see my spirit sparkling and alive,
my body healthy, divine and complete.
I see myself smiling and laughing, moving and dancing, feeling free.
I see my body at ease, delighting me deeply.
I can stay with these pictures as long as I please,
crystallising them lovingly in my mind's eye.
I can return to these pictures at any time I please,
seeing myself sparkling, and deeply at peace.

I take a few quiet moments to thank my body now.
My body that strives for me, and is there for me each day.
If there are any parts of me that I want to especially thank,
or perhaps especially encourage, I lovingly do so now.
When I feel ready, I gently open my eyes.
Breathing on with awareness,
I feel my body touched by my love.
Breathing in and out, I know my body loves me.

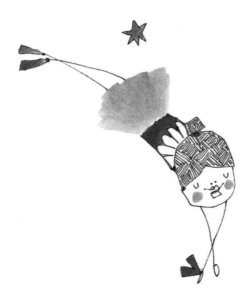

SELF-HEALING EXERCISES

Hippocrates, affectionately known as the father of modern medicine, famously pointed out that the doctor is not the one to heal the patient, but rather the one to awaken the natural healing powers within the patient themself. Indeed, we can awaken to our own healing powers and come to explore and cultivate a whole new part of our physical, emotional and spiritual intelligence.

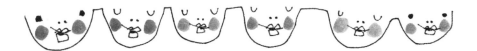

Have you ever noticed when you graze your knee, for instance, that the wound will heal on its own if the site is left clean and the body is left to do what it needs to do? We needn't interfere with our body's intelligence, nor must we control any process forcing our wound to repair. Very naturally and in perfect order blood clots to the site to suppress bleeding, a scab forms to protect the wound, and new skin regenerates in its place. This simple example manifests our body's profound ability to heal and regenerate, and demonstrates our body's 'knowingness' – a knowingness that cannot be learned, but that simply is.

Our bodies are inclined towards health when given half the chance. Our bodies embrace the faith we instil in them to heal. Optimising our conditions for wellbeing and self-healing is powerful preventative medicine. In his book *The Biology of Belief*, Dr Bruce Lipton delves into the riveting study of epigenetics: modern science proving that our lifestyles matter most, and that a healthy lifestyle can in many cases literally trump any genetic predisposition we may have to disease. It is fascinating to explore how our thoughts, beliefs and emotions affect and shape our health. Dr Lipton encourages us to see ourselves not as victims of our heredity but as powerful co-creators of our story, right at the helm of our wellness. Choosing to eat nourishing whole foods, prioritising rest and relaxation, moving our bodies and tending lovingly to our thoughts, we place ourselves and our bodies in prime position to flourish naturally, sparkle brightly and heal deeply.

These six simple self-healing exercises are ones that I draw on and hope you may enjoy. By no means should they take the place of any formal treatment protocol you may currently follow, while they may of course work in wonderful harmony with any such treatment to fortify, replenish and heal you, mind, body and spirit. Over time and with practice, you may just find these modes of self-healing boosting your general wellbeing and enhancing your immunity, allowing you to feel happier, healthier and more robust, even relying less on other forms of pain relief for which you might previously have reached. These simple techniques are right at our fingertips, supporting us to take loving care of our own needs, connect with our wonderful bodies and nurture our sparkles.

Breathing into Pain

When in pain, we often forget to breathe deeply. Deep breathing is a tonic for our nervous systems, minds and bodies. Breathing deeply and feeling life and energy flow fully into any area in which we feel pain can provide deep relief. Simply breathe in deeply and visualise your breath reaching the area of your pain, circulating it and gently creating spaciousness around it. As you inhale, flood that part of your body with breath, light and air. As you exhale, focus on the spaciousness you feel as you welcome more breath into that area. With each breath in and out, take your time. Focus your energy and attention carefully, and breathe on, as slowly and deeply as you can.

Talking to Pain

When I am in pain, I like to ask my body what it is trying to say to me. I allow myself to be guided, letting any pictures, words, memories or thoughts float in and out of my mind. If there is a conversation I need to have with myself, any person that needs forgiving, even if that person is me; if there is any old story I need to let go of or any special piece of wisdom from my spirit I am being called to acknowledge, I do so in this moment.

If nothing comes to mind or heart, I ask to be guided over the coming hours or day with a little healing hint or sign. We needn't hurry ourselves or force answers, as they will always come to us in perfect time. All we have to do is be self-compassionate, open to receiving healing, and deeply trusting in our ability to heal. Starting to enjoy conversations with our bodies can become a real pleasure. It is a form of self-love in motion, an ode to our sparkles. While this approach may be very new to you, even sound a little strange, I urge you to explore it. If you feel you'd like to, record any insights you receive in your diary. You may wish to use words, pictures or both to do so.

Loving Energy – Touch

In addition to breathing into our pain and conversing gently with it, we may also draw on our very own healing touch to bring relief and comfort to any part of our body. I always begin by gently rubbing my hands together and feeling the warmth and energy I can generate. Once I feel this warmth and energy I close my eyes and place my hands on the site of my pain. I hold my hands there, breathing into the site and focusing my attention upon it for as long as I feel comfortable. I might say 'thank you' or 'I love you' or 'I forgive you' as I touch the site of pain – any words that feel right. Sometimes such self-love can bring tears to my eyes. In this moment of surrender and release, I can sense healing happen and feel deep comfort. We all possess healing power in our hands. Our touch is very powerful. I encourage you to embrace and explore your own loving energy as you nurture your sparkle.

Focusing on Opposite Imagery

When I am in pain, I like to picture what that pain looks like. This helps me to make it seem less abstract and more material. If I have a headache for instance, I might visualise a very tight fist. This fist is held so tightly, the pressure is clenching and immense. I see this clenched fist in my mind's eye. Immediately after, I ask my mind to find an opposite for this image, say for instance an open palm. I see an open palm in my mind's eye, with light, air and space all around it. Holding these two images in my focus, I move between the clenched fist and the open palm, one after the other, breathing slowly and deeply in and out. I even like to clench and open my actual fist in unison with my visualisation to strengthen its effect. After a little while, I check in with the clenched fist. Suddenly it doesn't seem quite so tight. I use my mind in this way, flexing it with my attention until the pain I have been feeling begins to transform. This practice might take a little bit of getting used to, but it is a technique I find to be not only effective but deeply rewarding too.

Inviting the Divine Physician

Years ago it was suggested to me that I had a 'Divine Physician'. I had never heard of such a notion and was immediately very curious to explore it! I have since come to understand that in conjunction with our own healing energy work, we can call in our 'Divine Physicians' to perform little surgeries and energetically balance all manner of complex systems, from our digestion to our immunity and hormones, restoring our energetic bodies to their perfect blueprint. I now like to work together with my Divine Physician, asking for extra assistance and support when required. Like an added superpower, this is a wonderful energetic resource to engage in times of need. You might like to give your Divine Physician a name, a personality, even a specialty. Healing energy work can be as fun as we make it. Indeed, there is nothing quite like joy to help us heal.

Sending Light

Another simple way of working with healing energy is to visualise light within and around our bodies, cleansing, illuminating and refreshing us. We can let this healing light move through all our organs and cells, tissues and joints, muscles, blood and bones. We can let bright white light pulse in areas that feel painful or tense, assisting to relax and release them. We can send soft pink light around our hearts when we need extra emotional support and loving protection, and clear blue light to areas that feel overheated or inflamed. We can work intuitively with light and colour, sensing what feels most soothing, energising and healing to us at any given time. When we take the time to work together with our minds and bodies facilitating the healing we seek, we are deeply rewarded. We grow empowered by greater health, happiness and inner peace.

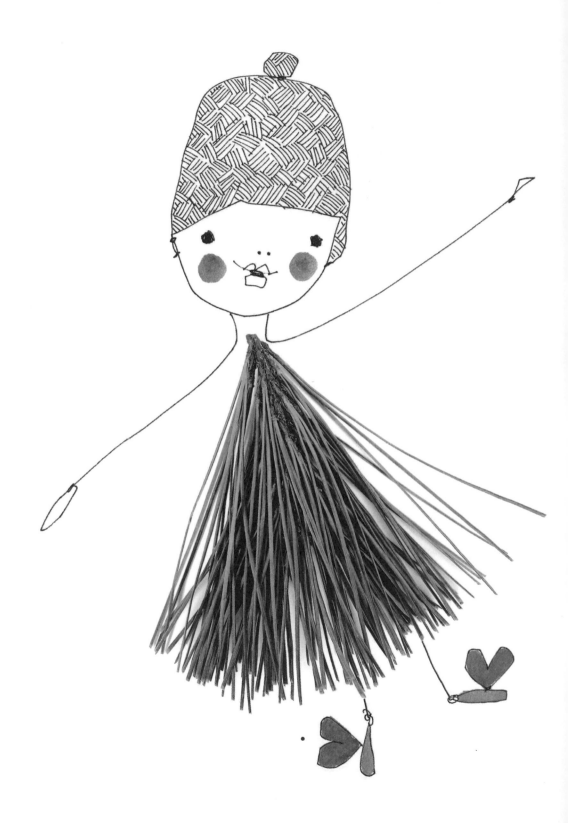

NATURE THERAPY FOR SPARKLING

Throughout these pages we have celebrated nature and the ways in which we can live in harmony with our earth, delighting, nurturing and nourishing our inner sparkles. Celebrating the idea that we can come home to ourselves and indeed heaven every time we reconnect with nature is a joy. Activities such as earthing, forest bathing, ocean bathing and even mindful sunbathing are nature's therapies, offering dazzling benefits that we may not even realise are freely available to us.

Quite simply, earthing involves placing our bare feet on the earth: the sand, the grass, the soil. A tremendously healing, grounding force of free electrons enters our bodies through the soles of our feet when we place them bare upon the earth. Indeed, the earth is our greatest, most fortifying and energising power source. Walking barefoot in your garden, at your local park, or along the sand at the beach are examples of earthing. Earthing ourselves as early as possible in the day helps to balance us mind, body and spirit, reconnecting us with ourselves and our world, with what is ancient, sacred and alive. Earthing is a wonderful, healthy counterpoint to the urban, technological spaces we often inhabit, disconnected from the power and presence of our earth. Studies have shown that earthing contributes to healing disease, relieving pain, decreasing inflammation and promoting restfulness and relaxation.

Forest bathing, known in the Japanese language as shinrin-yoku, literally means immersing ourselves amongst trees in nature. Studies have shown forest bathing to reduce stress, boost immunity, relax our physical bodies, promote feelings of wellbeing and even balance blood pressure. Fascinatingly, forest bathing expert Professor Yoshifumi Miyazaki cites studies in which those with high blood pressure showed a decrease in blood pressure when forest bathing, while those with low blood pressure saw an increase in blood pressure. Such findings demonstrate the profound, personalised and intuitive way nature brings each one of us back into balance. For those in close proximity to the wilderness, forest bathing is

a ritual to welcome more into your life. A day trip or weekend away into the trees might be just the ticket. Interestingly, for those lacking access to the wilderness, Professor Miyazaki has explained that similar effects to forest bathing may be garnered by touching and admiring flowers, or even a piece of wood. Such natural therapies are extraordinary, simple remedies to revive our sparkles.

The therapeutic benefits of submerging ourselves in luscious shades of green, the colour of vitality, helps to deeply soothe and re-energise us. Chlorophyll, the substance that makes plants appear green, is responsible for converting sunlight into energy. We too can feel energised by the experience of the colour green, and not just with our eyes. By eating our greens, as we are so strongly encouraged to do, we fortify ourselves with the tremendously stimulating and uplifting energy of light. We cannot forget that the energy of the sun, moon, wind and rain become part of us, filling us daily with new vitality.

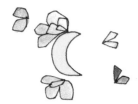

Ocean bathing is also renowned for its therapeutic effects. For many of us, swimming in the ocean has a healing effect upon our spirits, washing away our hurries and worries and instantly re-energising our sparkles. In addition to the mental and emotional benefits of such immersion, we know that saltwater can work wonders healing and restoring our skin. Being close to the ocean, walking barefoot along the shore and listening to the sound of waves roll in and roll out can be just as nourishing. The mind–body benefits of ocean therapy can be accounted for within the context of nature immersion, and the healing benefits of present-moment mindfulness. The feel of sand underfoot, the saltiness of the water and the rhythms of the waves catapult us into the present moment, connecting us with a vivid, inescapable sense of aliveness.

While ocean healing is something we can feel intuitively drawn to, it is being used in more structured contexts the world over now, playing a part in therapeutic programs supporting those with stress-related disorders such as PTSD (post-traumatic stress disorder), depression and low mood. Marine biologist Dr Wallace J Nichols explores this special topic in his wonderful book with a telling title: *Blue Mind: The surprising science that shows how being near, in, on, or under water can make you happier, healthier, more connected, and better at what you do.* If ocean therapy speaks to your spirit, this might be a wonderful book for you.

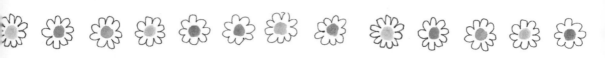

Mindful sunbathing is another natural way to energise and heal our bodies. Much fear around dangerous sun exposure has caused a deficiency in vitamin D that affects our bones, moods and more. While it is essential to inform ourselves about safe sun exposure, we needn't be terrified of the sun. Indeed, as my friend and Ayurvedic teacher Mark Bunn explains, sunshine can be healing for certain skin conditions such as rashes, cuts, infections, even eczema or psoriasis; it is wonderful for the prevention of physical disease, supportive of the health of our eyes, and essential for the lifting of our moods. In his book *Ancient Wisdom for Modern Health*, Mark recommends to greet the sun with gratitude and joy each morning, to seek some indirect early morning sunlight whenever possible to support general eye health, and at any time of the day to turn your face directly towards the sun with eyes closed. He suggests getting your vitamin D levels assessed, and better understanding the nature and ways of the sun to garner an appropriate level of exposure for you. Interestingly, dawn light is said to have a beneficial effect on our cognitive performance, making it all the more magical to rise joyously with the sun whenever possible.

Nature's remedies are powerful and simple. In addition to exploring the above activities for sparkle nourishment, commit as best as you can to honouring and harmonising with nature. In times gone by we rose with the sun and retreated with the moon. Our technological world with bright lights and screens of all kinds confuses our biorhythms, and many of us are missing the most precious, magical hours of sleep each night. These are the two hours before midnight, in which our bodies are perfectly attuned to detoxifying and restoring themselves.

Planning for early nights, switching off from overstimulating work and media after dark, and ensuring that we have a peaceful, well-ventilated and suitably dark sleeping space in which to rest all contribute to helping us sparkle more brightly in daily life. With a little care and by cultivating healthy, nourishing rhythms in our days, we can all become luminous morning stars!

Notice that nature allows seasons for all states of being: the extroversion and thrill of summer, the introversion and reflection of winter. As spring comes we are called to cleanse and refresh, and as autumn comes we are called to shed thoughts, ideas and things we no longer require, count the blessings from our summer harvest, and prepare ourselves for a more restful period. When we allow nature's wisdom to inspire our lives, we find a truly joyous, satisfying and sparkling sense of flow.

Nature-Inspired
Body Scan Meditation

I close my eyes and take a moment for myself now.
Closing my eyes and going within,
there is no place I would rather be. I take these quiet moments for myself,
breathing in and breathing out.

As I inhale I visualise my in-breath as a wave coming into shore.
Upon my exhalation, I see my out-breath a wave going out to sea.
With each breath in and out,
I feel waves coming in and gently going back out to sea.
From the soles of my feet right out through the top of my head,
I feel waves of breath flowing through my entire body now.
Breathing in, and breathing out.

When I feel ready I draw my attention to my abdomen,
visualising a fire burning bright within my belly.
I let this fire burn up any hurries or worries I may have,
any fears, doubts or negativity.
I visualise this fire like a glowing sun,
cleansing and illuminating my whole body.
I place my hands gently across my belly,
feeling it rise and fall. Breathing in and breathing out,
I feel the light and energy of my sun.

I draw my attention to my feet now.
I imagine walking my bare feet across soft grass.
Through soft sand, through crunchy autumn leaves.
As I breathe on, in and out, I let my feet potter.

When I feel ready, I draw attention to my hands.
I feel the softest sand between my fingers.
I sense my hands touch the trunk of an old tree.
I touch the delicate petals of a flower, one by one.

I spend a few moments with my hands now,
feeling each finger, feeling the palms and the back of my hands.
I feel the warmth of my hands, and sense the energy
within and around them.

When I feel ready, I hover the palms of my hands gently over my eyes.
I relax the spaces in and around my eyes,
breathing room into this area with each new inhale and exhale.
I imagine the space in and around my eyes expanding now,
as wide and deep as the night sky. Breathing on, I let this majestic night sky
take up as much room as it pleases.
Expanding. Boundless.

Sensing the magical energy of nature brimming within and around me now,
I slowly and gently open my eyes.

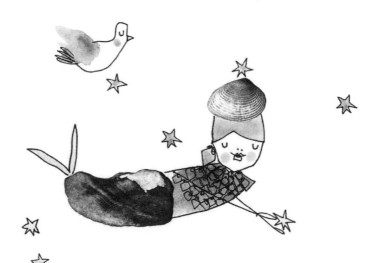

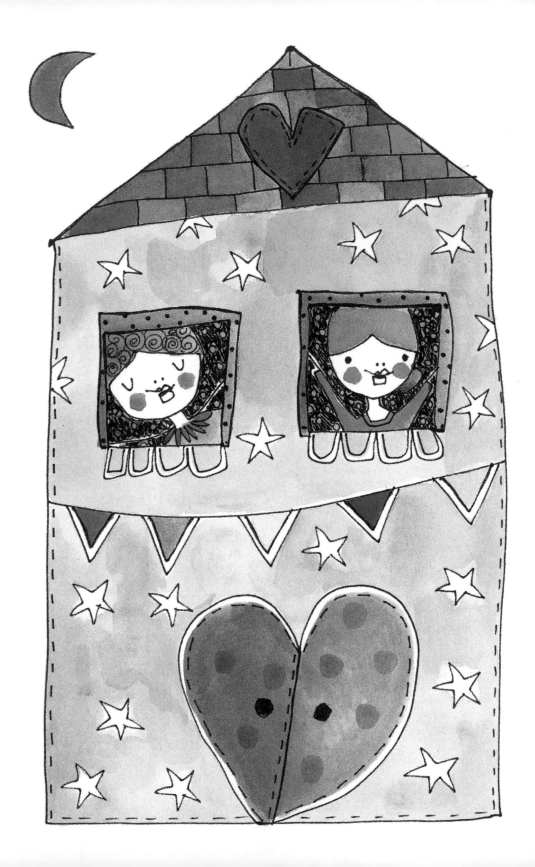

HOME CARE
FOR SPARKLING

I recently stumbled across a beautiful notion. If a flower isn't blooming, we don't fix the flower itself; we fix the conditions in which that flower is growing. Tending to our environments with loving energy is a gift we can grant ourselves each day. When we are in positive, uplifting and nurturing spaces our moods and mindsets are naturally elevated, lifting our complete sense of wellbeing. If we wish to sparkle, taking care of our surrounding environments and spaces will have magical effects.

While some of us are more sensitive to our environments than others, we all feel the energy of different spaces. Light, airy, clean and spacious places can elevate our spirits, beautiful gardens stir our souls, and thoughtful colours, scents and textures in spaces delight our senses. On the contrary, dark, untidy and unloved spaces can make us feel lacklustre, reduce our productivity and cloud our joy. In whatever ways we can, we are called to create beautiful spaces around us: spaces that elevate and inspire us and that contribute positively to our wellness, joy and peace.

I consider homes as our sanctuaries, sacred places in which to restore our spirits. While the world outside can be loud, bustling and beyond our control, our homes are our private retreats, special spaces that we can sculpt and savour. Choose a colour palette that nurtures and uplifts you. Select furniture, artwork and ornaments that inspire and delight you. Keeping your home neat and tidy and decluttering regularly will allow you to feel light and free in your space. I personally subscribe to the idea that less is more, choosing quality over quantity and keeping a simple, beautiful and peaceful home. I like to put things away as I use them, from shoes and clothes to teacups and books: a simple way to ensure a clear, relaxing flow within my home space.

Cleansing our homes with little rituals, sounds and scents can be truly soothing and energising. Some spaces carry heavy energy that can adversely affect our own.

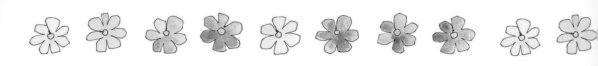

Even homes that lack ventilation or in which people have been arguing can carry an unsettled, burdensome air about them. If you are wishing to cleanse the energy in your home or simply want to uplift and refresh your sacred space, there are many simple, delightful options to explore. Open the windows and doors to allow light and air to circulate throughout your home. Try lighting a candle or some incense, arranging some fresh flowers or playing some blissful music. You may even like to try burning some sage or Palo Santo, cleansing and purifying botanicals traditionally called upon to cleanse and clear space. Placing stones, crystals and natural elements that resonate with you around your home can bring real vitality and healing power to your private sanctuary, supporting you to create a space in which you can feel nurtured, inspired and at peace.

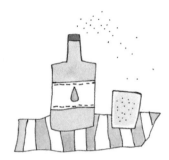

Tending to the cleanliness of our homes in natural ways is very important when it comes to nourishing our sparkles. Sadly, many home cleaning products are laden with health-tarnishing toxins and are quite unsafe for us to use and inhale. It is very hard to sparkle on when living amidst radiance-defying chemicals. You might find yourself with unexplained skin conditions, low moods, sinus-, allergy- and immune system–related concerns, not realising that your unclean cleaning products at home could be jeopardising your sparkling wellness. Detox your cleaning cupboard today, and explore the many inspiring, organic cleaning options now available to you.

You might even discover ways to make very simple, very effective cleaning products yourself using clean water, vinegar, pure essential oils of your choice, and basic bicarb soda. I guarantee that you will find DIY organic cleaning products more cost-effective, fun and exciting than supermarket varieties. In addition, the sense of peace and fulfilment you will feel in your naturally clean home will be more than worth the little effort it takes to get caring and creative in this clever way.

I love the idea of creating a sacred space at home, a special place in which we can stretch, meditate, go to think or decompress. This needn't be a big space; even a little corner will do. In this designated space I recommend placing objects, words, colours or inspirations of special significance to you, creating a little shrine to honour your peace and wellness, your health and happiness. This space can also be a communal sacred space if desired, created and enjoyed together by families. If any one person at any time is feeling the need to wind down, to retreat or regain perspective, they can approach this mutually respected place and know that they have a sacred space in which to feel healed, supported and nurtured at home. Creating a sacred space like this together, families can bring their joint attention to the spiritual life of each person within the home, and to the spirit of the home itself. Making the simple decision to create and look after a sacred space at home can be truly transformative.

It is very important that we remember to feel grateful for the spaces in which we live – to love and honour them daily. I like to look around my home and notice all the details. The way the light falls, and the various colours and textures I have chosen to adorn each room. I like to notice the creaks under certain floorboards, the birdsong beyond the window, the way wind tickles the windowpanes or the sound of rain on the roof. I savour pottering, cooking, cleaning, resting and relaxing at home, really allowing myself to feel nurtured, restored and supported by my space. Indeed, blessing our homes with our love, gratitude and mindfulness changes the way we feel about and exist within them.

Please enjoy the following blessing over your home, or be inspired to write and recite your very own. If you feel like writing the words of your home blessing down on paper, even embellishing them with drawings, pressed flowers or other beautiful details, you can create a special piece to be displayed in your home. I like the idea of finding a spot right at the front door, a place in which our blessings can be revisited and relished as we leave our nests, and again as we return home.

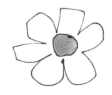

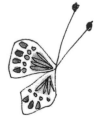

Home Blessing

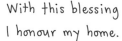

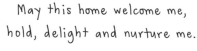

With this blessing
I honour my home.

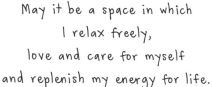
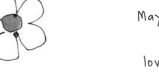

May this sacred space
be filled with light and joy,
peace and love.

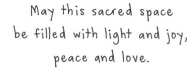
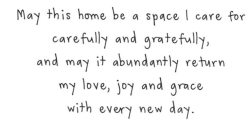

May this home welcome me,
hold, delight and nurture me.

May it be a space in which
I relax freely,
love and care for myself
and replenish my energy for life.

May this home be a space I care for
carefully and gratefully,
and may it abundantly return
my love, joy and grace
with every new day.

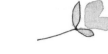

Family Home Blessing

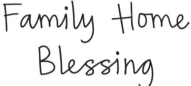

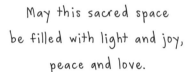

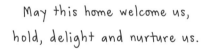

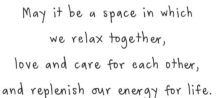

With this blessing
we honour our home.

May this sacred space
be filled with light and joy,
peace and love.

May this home welcome us,
hold, delight and nurture us.

May it be a space in which
we relax together,
love and care for each other,
and replenish our energy for life.

May this home be a space we care for
gratefully together,
and may it abundantly return
our love, joy and grace
with every new day.

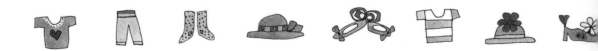

DRESSING TO SPARKLE

The old adage that 'clothes maketh the man' has always intrigued and delighted me. What's for sure is that we sparkle even more brightly, stand taller and feel better when we wear clothes that elevate and delight us. Dressing ourselves with care is a joyous part of daily life, and a creative way to nourish and express our unique sparkles.

The clothes and accessories we choose, the way we style our hair, the shoes we select and indeed the way we wear anything is expressive of our spirits. Our outer presentation is a representation of our inner world. Our self-presentation expresses our personalities, moods, ambitions and values, quite simply reflecting the way we see and feel about ourselves, and in part the way we wish others to see and know us too. While it goes without saying that what matters most is within us, presenting ourselves with love and care is part of honouring and celebrating our spirits. After all, our bodies are our spirit's gift-wrapping for life.

Dressing ourselves each day and enjoying colours, textures, shapes and styles that elevate and uplift us is a form of sparkle nourishment. When we feel beautiful and comfortable in our clothes it follows that we feel more confident and at ease in our day. We are all very different shapes and sizes, have differing preferences and varying activities that fill our days. Choosing clothes that suit and flatter us while allowing us to gracefully move our bodies through space is an art form. Even if simple, our clothes should make us feel wonderful. They should be joyous and effortless to wear, and express the love and care with which we honour ourselves.

We cannot underestimate the ways in which other people read us through our personal presentation, rightly or wrongly making all manner of assumptions about us based upon our clothing choices and personal grooming. At best, our outer style is congruent with our nourished inner sparkle, joyously expressing our love for ourselves and the delight we take in life.

Dressing and grooming ourselves with care, without fixating on our appearance, is not only a sign of our respect for ourselves, it is also an expression of our reverence for a sense of occasion in daily life. In my eyes, every day is worth celebrating. When we make the effort to present ourselves thoughtfully we bring a heightened sense of respect and appreciation to the various events, relationships, opportunities and pleasures life continually grants us to enjoy.

To help you look great, feel great and sparkle on each day, you might like to ask yourself the following questions when choosing your clothes daily or dressing yourself for a particular occasion. You might even like to explore them as journal prompts in your own quiet time.

What do these clothes say about me?

Does this feel true?

How do these clothes make me feel?

Do I enjoy feeling this way?

What does my personal grooming say about me?

Does this ring true for me?

In my clothes, I would like other people to see . . .

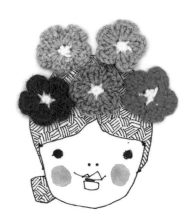

ESSENTIAL OILS AND CRYSTALS FOR SPARKLING

Essential oils and crystals are dazzling gifts from nature: magical resources drawn upon for their therapeutic benefits since ancient times. The materiality and energy of crystals connects us with our earth. Crystals sparkle with us, sharing the same fragments of stardust from which we too are created. Exploring the healing, protective and energising powers of essential oils and crystals can bring immense pleasure, comfort and sparkle into our daily lives.

As early as 3000 BC, Ancient Egyptians would add certain herbs and flowers to their baths, knowing them to offer therapeutic benefits. Botanical oils were transformed into medicines for health and healing, mummification and perfume. Ancient Egyptians were also renowned for using stones such as lapis lazuli, turquoise and carnelian in their jewellery to express status while also offering protection and health. Ancient Greeks and Romans would perform bathing rituals including scented oils, elevating the spirit through the nourishment of the physical body. While the healing benefits of essential oils and crystals are best understood intuitively, we can be guided by ancient wisdom around the power of certain essences and stones, exploring their ancient significance to touch our modern lives with magical energy.

STONES AND CRYSTALS

Stones and crystals are energetic compounds of natural elements, forming when liquids cool and start to harden. Stones and crystals are as ancient as our earth, dating back billions of years. They can be found within the crust of our earth, her rocks and soils. They appear to us in breathtaking formations and palettes of truly spectacular colour. What makes crystals so beautiful and mesmerising is the way light moves through them. We human beings are the same. When we welcome light into our lives, we sparkle. While all stones and crystals are sacred, as they derive from our earth, some are said to be imbued with particular magical powers.

Hematite

Said to be two billion years old, hematite is the most ancient mineral form of iron oxide. Often presenting in shimmering metallic grey, it may also appear in varied depths of muted red. Hematite is known to be a wonderful resource for energetic protection and, like black tourmaline, is used by many highly sensitive people, empaths and healers to help protect energetic boundaries and nurture the spirit.

Citrine

A light, warm and luminous quartz crystal, citrine is known to transmute negative energy, expand confidence and nourish creativity. I love to wear a beautiful citrine pendant around my neck. I certainly felt drawn to selecting this particular stone long ago, and still feel its magical essence every day.

Rose Quartz

Vitreous and translucent, rose quartz is a classic choice for drawing love and tenderness closer to us. It is a healing stone to support us when our hearts need a little bit of special love, when we need to embrace forgiveness of ourselves or others, or when seeking romance. When in need of extra loving energy I wear rose quartz jewellery, or place little pieces of rose quartz into my pockets and pillowslips.

Shungite

Black and lustrous, shungite is a wonderful, glossy mineral compound that, like graphite and diamonds, is mostly made of carbon. Shungite, said to have first been found in the village of Shunga in Russia, is appreciated to cleanse and purify energy. I like to place a piece of shungite on my desk and in my meter box at home, believing it to help diffuse strong electromagnetic frequencies. Shungite can also be placed at the bottom of water filters or jugs – not to be ingested, of course, but rather to facilitate the filtration and purification of drinking water. It is rumoured that Czar Peter (the Great), ruling over seventeenth- and eighteenth-century Russia, preferred to drink his water infused with shungite minerals.

Jade

Waxy and lustrous, jade is most known in its green and translucent presentation. Jade is a lovely choice for elevating our wellbeing as it is understood to soothe, uplift and clarify us. It is still honoured as a highly potent, precious and powerful stone in China today, where it has been a symbol of status, spirituality and purity for over nine thousand years. Jade (pounamou or greenstone) is also traditionally used and worn in Maori culture, with jade pendants representing ancestor spirits passed down from generation to generation along male lines. Jade is especially powerful when touching the body. You might like to explore jade jewellery, or find a set of jade prayer beads to touch during your meditations.

Clear Quartz and Amethyst

While there are a great number of crystals to explore, another two I particularly love and keep on hand are clear quartz, affectionately known by many as the 'master healer', and amethyst, the 'all-purpose stone'. Both these crystals are said to help clarify our thinking while bringing divine healing to our physical and energetic bodies. I enjoy the ritual of putting all my crystals out under a full moon to cleanse and energise them, and washing them in saltwater to purify them now and again. I like to add little crystals to my homemade body sprays, to my baths and water filter, wear them as jewellery and arrange them as objects of beauty around me.

ESSENTIAL OILS

Essential oils are the distilled essences of natural botanicals. There is a whole world of beautiful essential oils to explore, and to select in harmony with and support of our moods and needs. One of the most common ways to enjoy essential oils at home is through diffusers or oil burners, but there are many other ways that they can be savoured.

I personally apply a few drops of lavender oil to my wrists when feeling nervous or stressed, add a few drops onto my pillowslip or bath at night to ensure a more restful sleep, or into my washing for a beautiful fragrant result. I spray diluted lavender oil onto my curtains in summertime to keep mosquitoes at bay, and use it to soothe and heal insect bites and burns too.

As well as diffusing refreshing citrus oils such as lemon, lime, lemongrass and grapefruit for daily upliftment at home, I add them to my homemade cleaning products, room and body sprays. A big inhale of lemon oil can re-energise and refresh me from one moment to the next. I simply add a drop or two of lemon oil into the palms of my hands, rub them together, then breathe the scent deeply in, placing my hands lightly in front of my closed eyes. You might like to visit page 177 and be inspired to create delicious sweet biscuits infused with organic lemon oil!

Sandalwood is a particularly earthy and soulful essential oil. I love to rub a few drops of sandalwood oil into the soles of my feet at night, grounding and settling myself before bed. Sandalwood's anti-inflammatory, anti-viral properties also make it a great selection to boost immunity and fend off illness. The essential oil of cloves is an excellent choice for diluting and gargling to stop sore throats in their tracks, for application to pulse points in a carrier oil when travelling on aeroplanes or around people who are unwell, and for applying to the crown of the head and the soles of the feet in the presence of fever or malaise. Peppermint oil is energising and helps to clear our minds as well as our sinuses. When I have a cold or flu I add a few drops of peppermint oil to a tissue and inhale it deeply, or sprinkle it onto my pillowslip for easier breathing at night. I also add a drop of food-grade peppermint oil to my water glass or drink bottle for refreshment and to aid digestion, and clearing my sinuses all at once. A little peppermint oil in a carrier oil can be massaged into the temples when experiencing a headache.

This little handful of inspirations is just the beginning. Dip into the world of essential oils and crystals and prepare to be bedazzled! I always choose pure organic essential oils especially if ingesting them, and I am extremely careful with quantities and varieties, patch-testing if I'm planning to use them directly on my skin or in hand-crafted beauty products. It is advised that pregnant women or those with any health concerns at all seek advice before choosing and using essential oils at home.

Let's expand our awareness about nature's gifts, and enjoying a host of healing, soothing and sparkle-nourishing benefits in daily life.

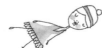 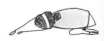

YOGA AND MEDITATION FOR SPARKLING

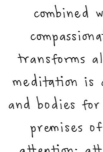

The ancient art of yoga is far more than physical stretches combined with mindful breathing. Yoga is an all-encompassing, compassionate and deeply spiritual way of life that touches and transforms all that we are and all that we do. Similarly, practising meditation is a time-honoured way to unite and harmonise our minds and bodies for sparkling health and happiness. The healing, restorative premises of both yoga and meditation are built upon our loving attention: attention to our bodies, our lives, and the world in which we live. When embraced in harmony, yoga and meditation can create a symphony of sparkle-nourishing benefits.

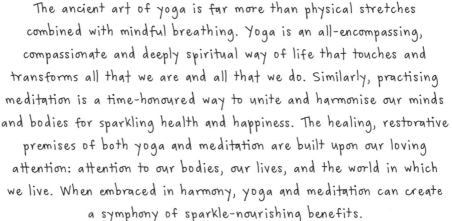

Mindfulness meditation involves bringing our attention to the present moment and is grounded in awareness of our breath: our life force. Following our breath we bring our minds to a full sense of our aliveness in the present moment, a practice that over time can imbue us with a sense of perspective, gratitude and deep inner peace. Meditation is scientifically proven to calm our nervous systems, helping us become more resilient to stress and anxiety, and gracing us with an expanded state of awareness, greater patience and increased overall vitality. The power of meditation is no secret. Indeed, the most successful people the world over attribute their tremendous performance, formidable energy levels and vibrant mental and physical health to its magic.

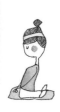
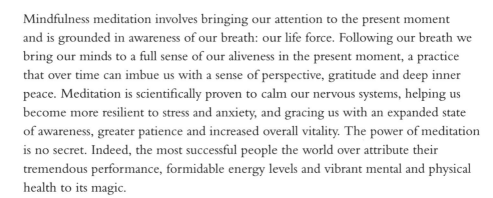

There are many wonderful ways in which we can explore meditation. We may like to begin our meditations by asking a question. We can then sit peacefully, simply with the intention of letting ideas and energy flow through us, providing us with deep insights, love and healing. Meditating upon a particular question is a simple, powerful way to connect more deeply with our intuition, and allow divine wisdom to arrive

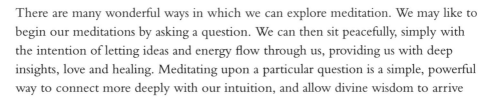

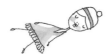   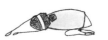

into our consciousness in perfect time. Meditating upon an affirmation or a mantra can also help us to strengthen and crystallise any thought we may wish to manifest. For example, if we are feeling stressed or strained, we may like to focus upon the word relax or calm. As we breathe in and out, we can hear the word of our choice repeated in our minds gently, over and over again. For some, certainly over the course of time, spoken or sung mantras have led to transcendental states: states in which departure from physical reality, time and space is felt and an entry into an expansive, boundless energetic realm is experienced. TM, or transcendental meditation, best describes this form of meditation in which mantra is often celebrated as a gateway to sublime and natural 'out of body' experiences.

While some of us may be drawn to a more formal practice of meditation, we might also find ourselves meditating in moving flow states while gardening, hand-crafting or performing any activity in which our mental attention is utterly focused while our minds and bodies are relaxed and at peace. We needn't be still, nor folded into a pretzel pose, to benefit from the art of meditation. The important thing to remember is that we simply cannot be bad at meditation; we can only be bad at finding time for it! Meditation is meant to be a joy, true nourishment for our sparkles. We can come to meditation with a sense of play or reverence, devotion or curiosity. However we come, we are called to open our hearts and minds. We are wise to remember that a tiny bit of meditation is better than none at all, and can even lead to a little bit more, and a little bit more beyond that!

If you would like to explore meditation further I offer a few simple suggestions to bring comfort and happiness to your practice. You may like to find a string of prayer beads with which to meditate. Prayer beads help to keep our hands busy and assist us to focus our attention. We might like to repeat our affirmation or mantra one time per bead, moving around our circle until complete. Prayer beads usually have a tassel along the line to mark our beginning and end point. If you like to meditate in a seated position, you might find yourself a beautiful, soft and comfortable cushion that supports you physically and allows you to feel as comfortable as possible throughout your meditation. Purpose-crafted meditation cushions can be found widely these days, or you may find the perfect cushion already existing somewhere around your home. I also highly recommend having a designated space in your home in which you can enjoy your meditations, imbuing this space with your special love and attention, and making it feel beautiful and sacred. You may like to bring a candle or some fresh flowers to this space, or any objects of beauty that enhance and elevate your meditation practice.

If you love to be outdoors in the fresh air and upon the earth's surface, meditating in nature can be a truly satisfying and sparkle-nourishing experience. You may enjoy the sound of waves rolling in and out, the song of birds in the trees around you, or the rustling of wind through the grass and the leaves. Add the extra element of earthing to your meditations and you'll no doubt sense truly magical benefits. If you wish to be reminded to meditate and would like extra support structuring your meditation practice, you may like to download various apps to your smartphone: apps with timers, reminders, and smorgasbords of guided meditations and visualisations are available to soothe and uplift you at any moment. A list of my favourite apps can be found in the 'Sparkling Resources' section of this book on page 228. You may also seek out meditation groups or classes in your local area for meeting like-minded people, learning new things and experiencing the tremendous energy of group meditation and collective consciousness.

I have personally practised yoga in conjunction with meditation since my early teens, and have found it to offer me a deep sense of inner peace and calm along with vital energy and greater physical, mental and emotional flexibility. My favourite form of yoga is Kundalini yoga, in which breath is very central to all parts of practice and in which I relish the flow of movement along with the joy of mantra and song. I love to practise yoga at home, even taking little breaks in my workday to replenish and revitalise myself with a series of poses and breathing sequences. While I most love to practise yoga by myself, I also enjoy attending yoga classes now and again to learn new things and connect with like-spirited people.

In the way of yoga for sparkling, I recommend starting your day with sun salutations. This special sequence of flowing movements honouring the sun engages and awakens the whole body, mind and spirit. Shoulder or head stands bring radiant beauty into our faces, helping to circulate blood and energy throughout our bodies, easing fatigue and anxiety, and supporting our immune systems. Holding bow pose in combination with the breath of fire, a light rhythmic breath that feels a little like sniffing, is a wonderfully strengthening, detoxifying combination that helps fortify our physical bodies while focusing our minds and cultivating mental and physical stamina. Cat and cow poses actively support the health of our glands. When practised one after the other in conjunction with the breath of fire, we help to nurture beautiful, happy and healthy bodies. It is both marvellous and miraculous how specific yoga poses can strengthen our external and internal physical bodies in various ways, from our muscles and joints to our bones and organs, while offering us the mental and emotional benefits of stress relief, deep relaxation and connection to our divine inner sparkles: the essence of sacred source energy within us. All things considered, yoga truly is a balm for lifelong radiance.

I love ending my days in the gentleness of child's pose or meditating in prayer pose: kneeling on the floor with my knees wide, my body stretched out in front of me, my forehead resting on the floor, arms extended and hands in prayer pose. I can stay in these deeply soothing poses for some time, tuning into my breathing while enjoying some beautiful, calming music to wind down.

Any time that I spend on my yoga mat feels like a commitment to myself: to the wellness of my spirit, my health and my happiness. Yoga is deeply loved and appreciated by so many around the world who practise it in all manner of ways each and every day. If yoga is something you are yet to explore I urge you to give it a try, experiencing for yourself the magical, comforting and sparkling energy it can cultivate within you.

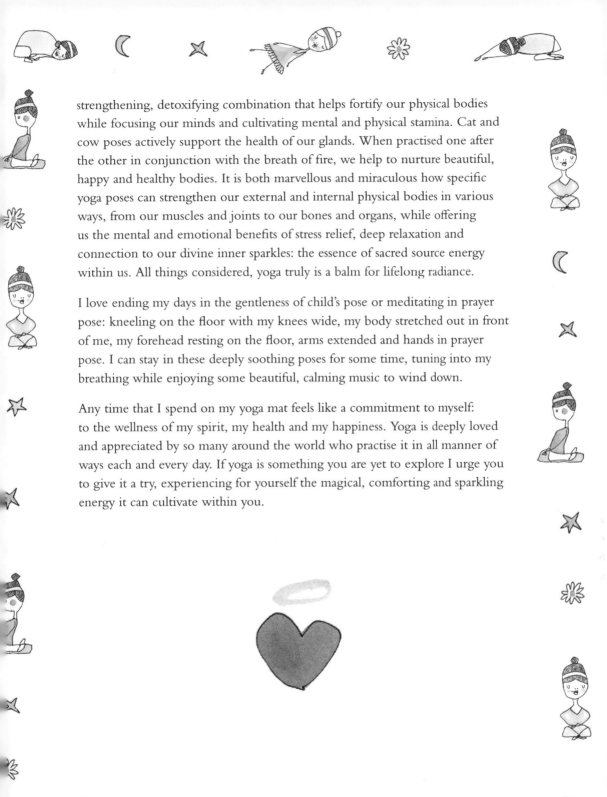

DEAREST YOU,

This is a book about exploring and nourishing your inner sparkle: your magic, wisdom, wilderness and wellness. When we nourish our sparkling spirits we feel alive. Our days naturally become more wonder-filled, meaningful and joyous, and we find ourselves balancing our inner and outer worlds with inspiration, wisdom and grace. Celebrating life means choosing not just to exist but to live. To answer the calls of our spirits and to create heavenly spaces within and around us.

Embracing the magic of life is very simple and joyous. This book has been created to encourage and motivate you as you choose to live with a sense of purpose and jubilation; as you face the patchwork of everyday life with its light, shade and in between; and as you seek not only just to exist but to live, fully – in every moment. When we are attuned to the vibrancy, creativity and freedom that is us and to the miraculousness of our existence on earth, we are deeply compelled to create lives far more than ordinary.

We all yearn to feel alive and loved, yet we feel lost and crestfallen when we seek our affirmation or rewards in the outer world: in others' approval, accolades or possessions. We miss so much when we look in all the wrong places, but we find so much when we seek our happiness within.

When we find, nurture and share our sparkles we contribute to the personal and collective meaning we seek. When we nourish our personal sparkle we join a collective energy nudging us closer to a happier, healthier and more peaceful world.

Beauty, peace and joy exist not somewhere out there, but within us. Once we find this sacred wellspring, this divine retreat within, we feel the relief and comfort for which we have been yearning. Lovingly releasing our hurries and worries, our doubts and fears, we may sparkle on with courage, faith and self-belief. All the seasons of our lives may be navigated with grace and savoured with joy simply by choosing to embrace the magic of life. When we live in day-to-day awareness of our luminous inner sparkles, infinite inspiration comes to us in all manner of subtle, enchanting and delightful ways. We can sharpen our wits to the miracles unfolding endlessly around us, and lead truly enchanted lives.

We have touched on self-care rituals, the value of community and connection, and the joy of living in contribution to a meaningful and magical bigger picture. We have explored ways in which we can all cultivate more sublime moments of tenderness, faith, surrender and bliss in daily life: ways in which we nurture ourselves deeply to sparkle from within. By choosing to find, accept and celebrate our divine sparkles, we naturally begin to see ourselves, each other and our world anew. We awaken to light, purpose and perspective, and replenish ever-new energy for life. We savour more wonderful moments than we could ever imagine.

May you feel inspired to find your sparkle right now, and to embrace the tremendous magic of life.

Until next time,

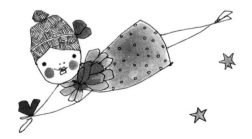

Love, Meredith X

Acknowledgements

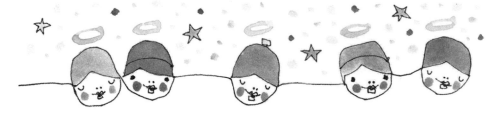

Finding, nurturing and nourishing my sparkle has been, and will continue to be, a lifelong journey of love, joy and inspiration. It would not be possible without the tremendous love and support of those with whom I share my life.

Firstly to my bedazzling husband, Mr Lindemann, whose sparkle utterly eclipsed me when we fell in love at first sight twelve years ago. Your constant care, your delightful sense of humour and zest for adventure tickle my spirit every day. You are so lovable, and so completely loved.

To my publisher, Pam Brewster, and her team at Hardie Grant in Melbourne including Jane Grant, Marg Bowman, my publicist Kirstie Armiger-Grant and the vibrant design crew, I thank you for your faith in me, your time, energy and support. I especially thank you, Pam, for inviting me to share my own sparkle with the world in this especially bountiful offering.

To the designer of this book and most of my other titles, creative angel Arielle Gamble, I thank you for your unending inspiration, attention to detail and care for my work. To Meaghan Thomson, I thank you for lovingly photographing my nature collages, and for preparing some of the digital conversions of my original watercolours that grace these pages. To Mick Smith and his team at Splitting Image, I thank you for handling so much of my artwork for publication. Your kindness and professionalism are always greatly appreciated.

To the wonderful editor of this book and several of my other books too, Allison Hiew, I thank you wholeheartedly for the grace, generosity and thoughtfulness with which you treat my words. You always let my voice be free while providing gentle nudges of encouragement and advice where needed. Thank you.

To my friends and family, you know who you are, I love and treasure you. To Tracy, Ivana, Michael, Mark and Nikki, you have taught me so much in friendship with your unique creativity and generous wisdom. Josette, your support within my business is treasured daily. Ian and Julie, Jeanette and Linda, I thank you very much for your constant counsel and care.

I lovingly dedicate this book to Kay Ridgway, my mountain mother and soul sister. My friend and confidante and the wisest, most sparkling spirit I have ever known. I love your love of life and your compassion for other human beings, the way you delight in nature — gardening and cooking with such care — your passion for meditation, qi-gong, and endless learning. I treasure the way we can natter unstoppably about the universe and our minds, bodies and spirits at the drop of a hat. I love how we share tea, stories and snippets of our lives together. I honour your radiance with this book, and present it to you with all my love.

Meredith X

SPARKLING RESOURCES

BOOKS

Daily Inspiration

101 Moments of Joy and Inspiration – Meredith Gaston
101 Inspirations for Your Journey – Meredith Gaston
A Course in Miracles Made Easy – Alan Cohen
A Deep Breath of Life – Alan Cohen
Essays and Poems by Ralph Waldo Emerson –
   Barnes & Noble Classic Series
The Little Prince – Antoine de Saint-Exupéry
The Prayer Tree – Michael Leunig
Rumi: The Book of Love – translation and commentary
   by Coleman Barks
Wabi Sabi: Japanese wisdom for a perfectly imperfect life –
   Beth Kempton
When I Talk to You – Michael Leunig

Self-Care

The Art of Extreme Self-Care – Cheryl Richardson
The Art of Gratitude – Meredith Gaston
The Art of Kindness – Meredith Gaston
The Beauty Guide – Dr Libby Weaver
Happiness: Essential Mindfulness Practices –
   Thich Nhat Hanh
*The Highly Sensitive Person: How to Thrive When the
   World Overwhelms You* – Elaine N. Aron, PhD.
Power Words: Igniting Your Life with Lightning Force –
   Sharon A. Klingler
You Can Heal Your Life – Louise Hay
You Were Not Born To Suffer – Blake D Bauer
Your Bed Loves You – Meredith Gaston
Your Sacred Self: Making the Decision to be Free –
   Wayne Dyer

Mind and Mindfulness

The Biology of Belief – Bruce Lipton
The Book of Tea – Kakuzo Okakurō
The Brain that Changes Itself – Norman Doidge
The Brain's Way of Healing – Norman Doidge
*Full Catastrophe Living: How to Cope with Stress, Pain and
   Illness Using Mindfulness Meditation* – Jon Kabat-Zinn

Happiness: Essential Mindfulness Practices –
   Thich Nhat Hanh
*Happy Genes: Tripping Your Inner Switches for Pleasure,
   Success and Relaxation* – Dawson Church
Ikigai: The Japanese Secret to a Long and Happy Life –
   Héctor García & Francesc Miralles
*Mind Over Meds: Know When Drugs Are Necessary,
   When Alternatives Are Better – and When to Let Your
   Body Heal on Its Own* – Dr Andrew Weil
No Mud, No Lotus – Thich Nhat Hanh
Optimism – Dawson Church
Peace of Mind – Thich Nhat Hanh
Soul Medicine – Dawson Church
Starbright Series: Meditations for Children –
   Maureen Garth

Wellness

Ancient Wisdom for Modern Health – Mark Bunn
The Art of Wellbeing – Meredith Gaston
*The Blue Mind: The Surprising Science That Shows How
   Being Near, In, On, or Under Water Can Make You
   Happier, Healthier, More Connected, and Better
   at What You Do* – Dr Wallace J Nichols
The China Study – T Colin Campbell &
   Thomas M Campbell
Elixir: How to Use Food as Medicine – Janella Purcell
The Genie in Your Genes – Dawson Church
GUT – Giulia Enders
*The Mind-Gut Connection: How the Hidden Conversation
   Within Our Bodies Impacts Our Mood, Our Choices, and
   Our Overall Health* – Dr Emeran Mayer
*Natural Health, Natural Medicine: The Complete Guide to
   Wellness and Self-care for Optimum Health* –
   Dr Andrew Weil
Nourishing Wisdom – Marc David
A Pukka Life – Sebastian Pole
Savor: Mindful Eating, Mindful Life – Thich Nhat Hanh
   & Lilian Wai-Yin Cheung
*Shinrin-yoku: The Japanese Way of Forest Bathing for
   Health and Relaxation* – Yoshifumi Miyazaki
Stressproof – Dr Mithu Storoni
The Tree of Yoga – BKS Iyengar

Women's Bodies, Women's Wisdom – Christiane
Northrup, M.D.
Women's Wellbeing Wisdom – Dr Libby Weaver
You Were Not Born to Suffer – Blake D Bauer
*Your Body's Many Cries for Water: You're Not Sick; You're
Thirsty – Don't Treat Thirst with Medications* –
Dr F. Batmanghelidj

Edible Nourishment

Bliss Bites – Kate Bradley
The Conscious Cook – Tal Ronnen
Crazy, Sexy Diet – Kris Carr
In Defense of Food: An Eater's Manifesto – Michael Pollan
Deliciously Ella Cookbooks – Ella Woodward
The Edible Balcony – Indira Naidoo
Ferment – Holly Davis
Green Kitchen Stories – Luise Vindahl
The Happy Pear: Recipes for Happiness –
David & Stephen Flynn
*Healing with Wholefoods: Asian Traditions and Modern
Nutrition* – Paul Pitchford
Kenkō Kitchen – Kate Bradley
My New Roots – Sarah Britton
Raw – Yoko Inoue
This Cheese is Nuts – Julie Piatt
Vegan Goodness – Jessica Prescott
Vegan 100 – Gaz Oakley

Creativity

21 Lessons for the 21st Century – Yuval Noah Harari
The Beauty of Everyday Things – Soetsu Yanagi
The Book of Tea – Okakura Kakuzō
The Creative License – Danny Gregory
How to be an Explorer of the World: Portable Life Museum
– Keri Smith
In Praise of Idleness – Bertrand Russell
The Leap Stories – Kylie Lewis
Messy Thrilling Life – Sabrina Ward Harrison
Real: Living a Balanced Life – Victoria Alexander
Sapiens: A Brief History of Humankind –
Yuval Noah Harari
Wabi-sabi for Artists, Designers, Poets & Philosophers –
Leonard Koren

Relationships

The Five Love Languages – Gary Chapman
Getting the Love You Want – Harville Hendrix
The Highly Sensitive Person in Love –
Elaine N. Aron, PhD
The Honeymoon Effect – Bruce Lipton

Decluttering and Slowing Down

Destination Simple – Brooke McAlary
*The Life Changing Art of Tidying Up: The Japanese
Art of De-cluttering and Organising* – Marie Kondo
The Minimalists – books by Joshua Fields Millburn &
Ryan Nicodemus
*The Minimalist Home: A Room-by-Room Guide
to a Decluttered, Refocused Life* – Joshua Becker
*The More of Less: Finding the Life You Want Under
Everything You Own* – Joshua Becker
In Praise of Slow – Carl Honoré
Slow: Live Life Simply – Brooke McAlary
*The Year of Less: How I Stopped Shopping, Gave Away
My Belongings, and Discovered Life is Worth More Than
Anything You Can Buy in a Store* – Cait Flanders

Our Earth

Earthing: The Most Important Health Discovery Ever? –
Clinton Ober, Stephen Sinatra & Martin Zucker
Grown and Gathered: Traditional Living Made Modern –
Matt & Lentil Purbrick
Healing our Planet, Healing Ourselves – Dawson Church
Mindfulness in the Garden – Zachiah Murray
Mindfulness and the Natural World – Claire Thompson
Second Nature: A Gardener's Education – Michael Pollan
We Are Here: Notes for Living on Earth – Oliver Jeffers

Energy and Magic

The 12 Stages of Healing – Donald M Epstein &
Nathaniel Altman
Anatomy of an Illness as Perceived by the Patient –
Norman Cousins
Compendium of Magical Things – Radleigh Valentine
The Crystal Bible – Judy Hall
Energy Medicine – Donna Eden & David Feinstein
Energy Medicine: The Scientific Basis –
James L Oschman PhD
Hands of Light – Barbara Brennan
Healing Myths, Healing Magic – Donald M. Epstein
*Practical Magic: A Beginner's Guide to Crystals, Horoscopes,
Psychics and Spells* – Nikki Van De Car
Spontaneous Evolution – Bruce Lipton &
Steve Bhaerman
*Spontaneous Healing: How to Discover and Embrace Your
Body's Natural Ability to Maintain and Heal Itself* –
Dr Andrew Weil
The Subtle Body – Cyndi Dale
You Are the Universe – Deepak Chopra &
Menas Kafatos

MAGAZINES

Breathe
Mindfood
Peppermint
Wellbeing
Womankind

WATCH

Bakara
Chasing Coral
The Chef's Table *Episode featuring Jeong Kwan
Consumed
The Cosmos
Cowspiracy
Dr Andrew Weil – 4-7-8 breathing technique, YouTube
Earth
Fed Up
Food Choices
Food Matters
Forks Over Knives
Global Waste
Happy
Heal
Human Planet
Hungry for Change
In Defense of Food
Made in Japan – BBC Scotland
The Minimalists
Plastic Oceans
Samsara
Seeds of Time
Sustainable
Terra
The True Cost
The War on Waste
What the Health
What the Bleep Do We Know

LISTEN

Buddhify (app)
Calm (app)
The Deliciously Ella Podcast
Hay House Radio (podcast)
Hay House World Summit (podcast)
Headspace (app)
Insight Timer (app)
Jon Kabat-Zinn Mindfulness Meditation Tapes
Louise Hay Affirmations and Lectures
The Mind Body Green Podcast
Mindful Kind podcast – Rachael Kable
The Minimalists Podcast
Ofkin Podcast
Oprah's SuperSoul Conversation Podcasts
The Rich Roll Podcast
Slow Your Home (podcast)
Smiling Mind (app)
Stephen Cabral Podcast

VISIT

www.biome.com.au
www.blackchicken.com.au
www.catherinecollautt.com
www.thedailyguru.com
www.dawsonchurch.com
www.deliciouslyella.com
www.drhyman.com
www.greenkitchenstories.com
www.hayhouse.com
www.inikacosmetics.com.au
www.kriscarr.com
www.leunig.com
www.meredithgaston.com
www.mindbodygreen.com
www.theminimalists.com
www.mynewroots.org
www.ofkin.com
www.ted.com
www.truecostmovie.com

FITNESS

Jessica Smith TV (www.jessicasmithtv.com)
Raviana: Kundalini Yoga (www.raviana.com)
Ballet Beautiful (www.balletbeautiful.com)